Health Lessons

by Alvin Davison

PREFACE

Scarcely one half of the children of our country continue in school much beyond the fifth grade. It is important, therefore, that so far as possible the knowledge which has most to do with human welfare should be presented in the early years of school life.

Fisher, Metchnikoff, Sedgwick, and others have shown that the health of a people influences the prosperity and happiness of a nation more than any other one thing. The highest patriotism is therefore the conservation of health. The seven hundred thousand lives annually destroyed by infectious diseases and the million other serious cases of sickness from contagious maladies, with all their attendant suffering, are largely sacrifices on the altar of ignorance. The loving mother menaces the life of her babe by feeding it milk with a germ content nearly half as great as that of sewage, the anemic girl sleeps with fast-closed windows, wondering in the morning why she feels so lifeless, and the one-time vigorous boy goes to a consumptive's early grave, because they did not know (what every school ought to teach) the way to health.

Doctor Price, the Secretary of the State Board of Health of Maryland, recently said before the American Public Health Association that the text-books of our schools show a marked disregard for the urgent problems which enter our daily life, such as the prevention of tuberculosis, typhoid fever, and acute infectious diseases.

Since the observing public have seen educated communities decrease their death rate from typhoid fever, tuberculosis, and diphtheria from one third to three fourths by heeding the health call, lawmakers are becoming convinced that the needless waste of human life should be stopped. Michigan has already decreed that every school child shall be taught the cause and prevention of the communicable diseases, and several other states are contemplating like action. This book meets fully the demands of all such laws as are contemplated, and presents the important truths not by dogmatic assertion, but by citing specific facts appealing to the child mind in such a way as to make a lasting impression.

After the eleventh year of age, the first cause of death among school children is tuberculosis. The chief aim of the author has been to show the child the sure way of preventing this disease and others of like nature, and to establish an undying faith in the motto of Pasteur, "It is within the power of man to rid himself of every parasitic disease."

Nearly all of the illustrations used are from photographs and drawings specially prepared for this book. These, together with the large amount of material gleaned from original sources and from the author's experiments in the laboratory, will, it is hoped, make this little volume worthy of the same generous welcome accorded the two earlier books of this series.

CONTENTS

HEALTH LESSONS

CHAPTER I

CARING FOR THE HEALTH

=Good Health better than Gold.=--Horses and houses, balls and dolls, and much else that people think they want to make them happy can be bought with money. The one thing which is worth more than all else cannot be bought with even a houseful of gold. This thing is good health. Over three million persons in our country are now sick, and many of them are suffering much pain. Some of them would give all the money they have to gain once more the good health which the poorest may usually enjoy by right living day by day.

=How long shall you live?=--In this country most of the persons born live to be over forty years of age, and some live more than one hundred years. A hundred years ago most persons died before the age of thirty-five years. In London three hundred years ago only about one half of those born reached the age of twenty-five years. Scarcely one half of the people in India to-day live beyond the age of twenty-five years. In fact, people in India are dying nearly twice as fast as in our own country. This is because they have not learned how to take care of the body in India so well as we have.

The study which tells how to keep well is Hygiene. Whether you keep well and live long, or suffer much from headaches, cold, and other sickness, depends largely on how you care for your body.

=Working together for Health.=--One cannot always keep well and strong by his own efforts. The grocer and milkman may sell to you bad food, the town may furnish impure water, churches and schools may injure your health by failing to supply fresh air in their buildings. More than a hundred thousand people were made very sick last year through the use of water poisoned by waste matter which other persons carelessly let reach the streams and wells. Many of the sick died of the fever caused by this water. Although it cannot be said that we are engaged in real war, yet we are surely killing one another by our thoughtless habits in scattering disease. We must therefore not only know how to care for our own bodies, but teach all to help one another to keep well.

=A Lesson from War.=--The mention of war makes those who know its terrors shudder. Disease has caused more than ten times as much suffering and death as war with its harvest of mangled bodies, shattered limbs, and blinded eyes. In our four months' war with Spain in 1898 only 268 soldiers were killed in battle, while nearly 4000 brave men died from disease. We lost more than ten men by disease to every one killed by bullets.

In the late war between Japan and Russia the Japanese soldiers cared for their health so carefully that only one fourth as many died from disease as perished in battle. This shows that with care for the health the small men of Japan saved themselves from disease, and thus won a victory told around the world.

=The Battle with Disease.=--For long ages sickness has caused more sorrow, misery, and death than famine, war, and wild beasts. Many years ago a plague called the black death swept over most of the earth, and killed nearly one third of the inhabitants. A little more than a hundred years ago yellow fever killed thousands of people in Philadelphia and New York in a few weeks. When Boston was a city with a population of 11,000, more than one half of the persons had smallpox in one year. Within a few years one half of the sturdy red men of our forests were slain by smallpox when it first visited our shores. Before the year 1798 few boys or girls reached the age of twenty years without a pit-marked face due to the dreadful disease of smallpox. This disease was formerly more common than measles and chicken pox now are because we had not yet learned how to prevent it as we do to-day.

=Victory over Disease.=--Cholera, yellow fever, black death, and smallpox no longer cause people to flee into the wilderness to escape them when they occasionally break out in a town or city. We have learned how to prevent these ailments among people who will obey the laws of health.

Until the year 1900, people fled from a city when yellow fever was announced, but now any one can sleep with a fever patient and not catch the disease, because we have learned how to prevent it. Nurses and doctors no longer hesitate to sit for hours in the rooms of those sick with smallpox because they know how to treat the body to keep away this disease. By studying this book, boys and girls may learn not only how to keep free from these diseases, but how to manage their bodies to make them strong enough to escape other diseases.

=As the Twig is bent so the Tree is inclined.=--This old saying means that a strong, straight, healthy, full-grown tree cannot come from a weak and bent young tree. Health in manhood and womanhood depends on how the health is cared for in childhood. The foundation for disease is often laid during school years. The making of strong bodies that will live joyous lives for long years must begin in boyhood and girlhood.

In youth is the time to begin right living. Bad habits formed in early life often cause much sorrow in later years. It is said that over one half the drunkards began drinking liquor before they were twenty years of age and most of the smokers began to use tobacco before they were twenty years old.

PRACTICAL QUESTIONS

1. What is worth most in this world?

2. How many people are sick in our country?

3. How long do most people live?

4. Why do people not live long in India?

5. What is hygiene?

6. How many more deaths are caused by disease than by war?

7. Give some facts about smallpox.

8. Why do we have no fear of yellow fever and smallpox now?

9. Why should you be careful of your health while young?

10. When do most smokers and drinkers begin their bad habits?

CHAPTER II

PARTS OF THE BODY

=Regions of the Body.=--In order to talk about any part of the body it must have a name. The main portion of the body is called the trunk. At the top of the trunk is the head. The arms and legs are known as limbs or extremities. The part of the arm between the elbow and wrist is the forearm. The thigh is the part of the leg between the knee and hip.

The upper part of the trunk is called the chest and is encircled by the ribs. The lower part of the trunk is named the abdomen. A large cavity within the chest contains the lungs and heart. The cavity of the abdomen is filled with the liver, stomach, food tube, and other working parts.

=The Plan of the Body.=--All parts of the body are not the same. One part has one kind of work to do while another performs quite a different duty. The covering of the body is the skin. Beneath is the red meat called muscle. It looks just like the beef bought at the butcher shop which is the muscle of a cow or ox. Nearly one half of the weight of the body is made of muscle.

The muscle is fastened to the bones which support the body and give it stiffness. The muscle by pulling on the bones helps the body to do all kinds of work. The muscles and bones cannot work day after day without being fed. For this reason a food tube leads from the mouth down into the trunk to prepare milk, meat, bread, or other food, for the use of the body.

=Feeding the Body.=--The mouth receives the food and chews it so that it may be easily swallowed. It then goes into a sac called the stomach. Here the hard parts are broken up into tiny bits and float about in a watery fluid. This goes out of the stomach into a long crooked tube, the intestine. Here the particles are made still finer, and the whole mass is then ready to be carried to every part of the muscles, bones, and brain to build up what is being worn out in work and play.

=Carrying Food through the Body.=--In all parts of the body are little branching tubes. These unite into larger tubes leading to the heart. Through these tubes flows blood. Hundreds of tiny tubes in the walls of the intestine drink in the watery food, and it flows with the blood to the heart. The heart then pushes this blood with its food out through another set of tubes which divide into fine branches as they lead to every part of the body (Fig. 5).

=Getting rid of Ashes and Worn-out Parts.=--The body works like a machine. Food is used somewhat as a locomotive uses coal to give it power to work. Some ashes are left from the used food, and other waste matter is formed by the dead and worn-out parts of the body. This waste is gathered up by the richly branching blood tubes and carried to the lungs. Here some of it passes out at every breath. Part of the waste goes out through the skin with the sweat and part passes out through the kidneys. In this way the dead matter is kept from collecting in the body and clogging its parts.

=How the Parts of the Body are made to work Together.=--The mass of red flesh covering the bones is made up of many pieces called muscles. Whenever we catch a ball or run or even speak, more than a dozen muscles must be made to act together just in the right way. When food goes into the stomach, something must tell the juice to flow out of the walls to act on the food. The boss or manager of all the work carried on by the thousands of parts of the body is known as the brain and spinal cord with their tiny threads, the nerves, spreading everywhere through bones and muscles. The brain and spinal cord give the orders and the nerves carry them (Fig. 5).

=The Servants of the Body.=--The parts of the body are much like the servants in a large house or the clerks in a store. One servant or clerk does one kind of work while another does something entirely different. Each portion of the body does a different kind of work. Each one of these parts doing a particular work is called an organ. The stomach is an organ to prepare food and the heart is an organ for sending the blood through the body.

The entire body is composed of several hundred organs. Each of them is formed of several kinds of materials named tissue. A skinlike tissue makes up the lining of the stomach, while its outside is made of muscular tissue. The smallest parts of a tissue are little bodies named cells, and very fine threads called fibers.

=Growth of the Body.=--The body grows rapidly in childhood and more slowly after the sixteenth year, but it continues to get larger until about the twenty-fifth year of age. Some children always grow slowly, have weak bones, and frail bodies. This is generally so because they have poor food or do not chew it well, and get too little fresh air, sunshine, and sleep.

The use of beer, wine, or tobacco may hinder the body from using food for growth, or they may poison the body so that it will never be large and strong. The body should grow about a hundred pounds in weight during the first thirteen years of life. Whether children grow little or much generally depends on the food they give their bodies.

PRACTICAL QUESTIONS

1. Point out and name four parts of the body.

2. Name the two parts of the trunk.

3. What does the chest contain?

4. What is muscle?

5. How is the body fed?

6. Give three parts taking waste out of the body.

7. Of what use are the brain and nerves?

8. Name two organs.

9. How long does the body continue to grow?

10. Why are some children weak and of slow growth?

CHAPTER III

FEEDING THE BODY

=Why the Body needs Food.=--Every living thing, whether a plant or an animal, needs food. While the whole body lives, a part of it is constantly dying.

The entire outer layer of a snake's skin dies three or four times during a year and is cast off, sometimes in a single piece. We can scrape dead bits of skin from the surface of our body at any time. Tiny particles are dying in all regions of the body, and we should soon waste away if food were not taken to make up the loss for the worn-out parts.

The body also needs food to help it do its work and keep warm. The body has the strange power of using food eaten to make the legs and arms move and the brain to think. In doing this the body is said to burn the food.

=How the Body burns itself and also Food.=--If a boy is weighed just before playing a game of ball and again afterward, he will find that part of his body has been used up and given off in the breath and sweat. He has burned part of his body, and the breath and sweat are like the smoke given off when a match is burned.

One fifth of the air is made of a gas called oxygen. When anything becomes very hot, this oxygen makes it burst into a flame and burn. We breathe in oxygen with the air and the living action of the body causes such a slow union of the oxygen and the tissues that there is no blaze although there is a little heat.

=Kinds of Food.=--There are four general classes of foods. These are the building foods, the sugars and starches, the fats, and the mineral foods. The building foods are those which help largely in forming new muscle and blood or other parts of the body. Proteids is another name for building foods.

Sugars and starches are placed in one group because starch changes to sugar within the body. If you chew a starchy food like bread for a few minutes, it will begin to taste sweet because the starch is becoming sugar.

Fats are got not only from fat meat but also from eggs, butter, milk, and many other foods. There is some mineral matter, such as potash and soda, in many of the vegetables and meats eaten, and we use much table salt to season other foods.

=Body-building Foods.=--A person with all the sugar, molasses, starch, butter, and lard he could eat would starve to death in a few weeks because none of these foods would help to build up the dying parts of the body. A large amount of body builder is found in lean meat, eggs, milk, peas, beans, corn meal, and bread. Bread and milk is a good food to make the body grow. If the body takes in more building food than it needs for repairs, it may store it up in the form of fat or burn it to help the body do its work.

=The Fuel Foods.=---The fuel foods are the sugars, starches, and fats. These are the foods which the body can easily burn to keep it warm and give it power to act. Candy, molasses, or sugar in any form, taken in small quantities, is a good food. Starch, which the body quickly changes to sugar, is a much cheaper food. Meats contain very little starch, but nearly all vegetables contain much starch. Three fourths of corn meal, rice, wheat flour, and soda crackers consists of starch. More than one half of white bread, dried beans, and peas is made of pure starch, and there is much starch in potatoes.

Fat is more abundant in animal than in vegetable food. Castor oil and cotton-seed oil are fats from vegetables. The fat of the cow is called suet or tallow, while the fat of the hog is known as lard. Butter is the fat collected from milk. Cream and eggs contain much fat. When persons eat too much of the sugars, starches, or fats, the body may store them up as fat. For this reason thin persons wishing to gain in flesh eat eggs, nuts, and rich milk.

=The Mineral Foods.=---The body must have not only lime to help form the bones, but iron, salt, soda, and potash for other parts of the body. All these minerals except salt are found in many of the common foods.

Water is one of the most important of the mineral foods because it helps the body use all the other foods. Most people drink too little water to enjoy the best health. The body needs more than two quarts of water every day. There is much water in our foods. More than one half of eggs, meat, and potatoes is made of water, and more than three fourths of tomatoes, green corn, onions, cabbage, and string beans is composed of water. We should drink one quart or more of water daily. It should not be used ice cold, and very little should be taken at meal time.

=Water and Health.=---One of the common causes of sickness is bad water. Water from shallow wells within a hundred feet of barnyards, pigpens, or other outhouses is usually unsafe to drink. At Newport, Rhode Island, more than eighty persons were made sick with the fever by drinking the water from a well only ten feet deep. The impure water from one spring at Trenton, New Jersey, gave the fever to nearly a hundred persons in one season. At Mount Savage, Maryland, a hundred and twenty persons were made ill by using the water from a spring near a house drain.

Water from rivers and streams running near where many people live is likely to be made impure and is sure to bring sickness and death to some of those who use it. Water from a small stream at Plymouth, Pennsylvania, running past a house occupied by a typhoid patient, gave the fever to over a thousand persons in one month. The water from a small stream at Ithaca, New York, gave the fever to over thirteen hundred people in one season, and an almost equal number caught the fever in a few weeks at Butler, Pennsylvania, by drinking water from a small creek along which some sick persons lived.

=Preventing Sickness from Bad Water.=--It is better to go thirsty than to drink water which is likely to cause sickness. Any water can be made safe by boiling it one minute. Boiled water is the most healthful kind of water to use. The people of China and Japan seldom use water that has not been boiled.

Many cities using water from rivers run it through a layer of sand and gravel to remove the tiny things that cause so much sickness and death. This makes the water very much purer, but it is not so certain to make the water safe as is boiling it. Bad water makes nearly a quarter of a million of our people sick every year and kills twenty thousand of them.

=How much Food does the Body Need?=--Most people eat too much. Overeating overworks the stomach, poisons the body, makes one feel lazy, and causes headache. If you chew your food fine and stop eating as soon as hunger is satisfied without tempting the appetite with sweets, you are not likely to overeat.

About one seventh of a pound of building food is needed daily to keep the body in repair, and a quarter of a pound of fat and a pound of starches and sugars are required to help the body do a hard day's work. A half pound of bread, beans, and meat each, a pound of potatoes, a pint of milk, and a quarter of a pound of butter and sugar each, will give a working man all the food he needs for a day.

=Beer and Wine as Foods.=--It was once thought that beer and wine were good foods, but hundreds of late experiments show that these drinks are very poor and expensive foods. A half glass of milk is of more use to the body as a food than a full quart of beer. The use of much wine or beer may seem to satisfy the appetite because they deaden the real feeling of hunger. Neither of these drinks can be used by the young without danger of doing much harm.

PRACTICAL QUESTIONS

1. Why does the body need food?

2. Why do you weigh less after working?

3. What is oxygen?

4. From what do we get body-building foods?

5. In what is starch found?

6. How much water does the body need?

7. Where have people been made sick by using bad water?

8. How can we prevent sickness from bad water?

9. What harm does overeating do?

10. What can you say of beer as a food?

CHAPTER IV

FOOD AND HEALTH

=Meats.=--Beef is the best of all meat for food. Nearly one fifth of it can be used to repair the worn-out parts of the body. Mutton, the meat of sheep, is almost as good for food as beef. Veal and pork also contain much body-building matter, but the stomach must work hard to prepare them for use.

Fish is an excellent food, but it has only little more than one half as much flesh-building matter as good beef. Poultry is a healthful food, especially for the weak and sick, but it is more expensive than the other meats. Oysters are largely made of water and do not contain much to strengthen the body.

In all meat there is some waste matter. This may harm the body if we eat too much meat. It is no longer thought healthful for most persons to eat meat more than once a day. Too much meat used daily for several years is likely to cause disease.

=The Cooking of Meat.=--The best meat if poorly cooked is unfit for eating. Broiled and roasted meats are more healthful than boiled or fried meat. Meat is broiled by holding it in a wire frame over a flame or hot coals. It is roasted by placing it in a covered pan in a hot oven for two or three hours. It is boiled by keeping it in hot water several hours.

Meat is fried by cooking it in lard or other fat in a pan. Only those who have strong bodies should eat fried meat.

The cheap cuts of meat from the neck, breast, and legs have about as much food matter in them as the more costly parts. Such meat may be made more tender by boiling than by roasting.

=Soup.=--Soup, broth, and beef tea furnish but little food for the body. They are very useful in giving us a good appetite for the real food to be eaten later. They make the stomach go to work more quickly than other food. Soup or broth is made from meat by placing it on the stove in cold water, gradually heating it, and then keeping it hot several hours.

=Vegetables.=--Some persons never eat meat of any kind because they enjoy better health when using only vegetables, milk, and eggs. Peas and beans contain much matter for making new flesh and blood and also much starch to give heat and power to the body. Potatoes form a valuable food. Roasted potatoes are more healthful than those boiled or fried.

Radishes, onions, and cucumbers are made largely of water. Only a small amount of these should be eaten at one meal as the stomach must work hard to make use of them. Young beets, lettuce, and ripe tomatoes may be eaten by young and old. They contain useful minerals and help keep the body in a healthful condition.

=The Cereals or Grain Foods.=--These foods are eaten in the form of bread, oatmeal, corn meal, rice, and breakfast foods. All of these furnish much matter to strengthen the body and make it grow. Bread and butter with rice are excellent foods for children.

=Fruits.=--Very few people can remain well long without eating fruit of some kind. Ripe apples, pears, plums, peaches, berries, and cherries furnish useful salts to the body and also help the stomach and food tube do their work in a more healthful way. Fruits also increase the appetite. Green fruit and fruit which is overripe should never be eaten.

=Eggs.=--Eggs form a good food for nearly everybody, but they are specially needed by the young and other persons with weak bodies. They can repair the worn-out parts of the body and also help it do its work.

Eggs are most healthful when eaten raw or soft cooked. The best way to cook them through evenly is to put them in a pan off the stove and add about a quart of boiling water for every three eggs. Cover and let them cook fifteen minutes.

Eggs should be kept in a cold room or cellar until used. They become stale in less than a week when left in a warm living room and may get a bad taste when only three or four days old.

=Salt, Pepper, and Vinegar.=--Eating much salt is harmful. A small quantity of salt and pepper increases the appetite and makes the stomach do its work better. Children should use very little pepper and almost no vinegar and mustard.

=Tobacco.=--Some people think tobacco is a food because it is made from the leaves of a plant. Other people think tobacco is a food because they do not feel hungry after smoking or chewing it. The truth is that tobacco is of no use to the body as a food and may do it much harm because of the poison it contains. Tobacco satisfies hunger somewhat by deadening the parts of the body that are calling for food.

=Beer.=--The people who make beer and sell it say that it is a food. Men who have no interest in selling beer, and have experimented with it to find out whether it strengthens the body, say that beer should never be used as a food. It often tends to weaken the body. Children should never use beer at any time, and older people can sometimes avoid disease by letting it alone.

PRACTICAL QUESTIONS

1. Which are the best meats for food?

2. Why should we not eat meat at every meal?

3. How should meat be cooked to make it most tender?

4. How is soup or broth made?

5. Name the best vegetables for food.

6. Name some good grain foods.

7. Of what use are fruits?

8. What can you say of the use of eggs?

9. How should eggs be cared for?

10. What can you say of the use of salt and pepper?

11. Why does tobacco satisfy hunger?

12. Of what value is beer for food?

CHAPTER V

HOW PLANTS SOUR OR SPOIL FOOD

=Germs, Microbes, or Bacteria.=--The dust and dirt of all sorts contain thousands of tiny plants too small to be seen by the eye without help. An instrument called a microscope makes them appear so large that their form and growth are easily studied. These little plants are called germs or microbes. They are also named bacteria. They are so small that a million laid side by side would not cover the head of a pin.

There are hundreds of different kinds of germs. Some are round like little balls and others are the shape of tiny rods. Many of them which look just alike act very different in growing. There are more than twenty different kinds that grow in our bodies and cause diphtheria, tuberculosis, and other diseases. We have measles and scarlet fever because we have gotten these disease germs from some one else in whom they were growing.

Most germs feed on dead matter instead of our living bodies and make it melt away or change into another form. An apple or a piece of meat thrown out on the ground will soon change and become like the earth on which it lies. The change, called decay, is caused by millions of germs. The farmer's best friends are certain germs which help make the ground rich, so that the crops will grow.

=Mold.=--The dust raised in sweeping contains tiny living seedlike bodies. If these fall on bread, cheese, or fruit, and this food is afterward kept moist in a warm room for a day or two, they will grow into grayish fluffy spots. These spots are mold. The greenish white growth on the top of some canned fruit and on berries left in the warm kitchen over night is also mold.

Mold is a plant which grows from tiny round bodies acting like seeds (Fig. 17). These seed bodies of mold are common in all dust and often fly through the air. On this account food should be kept covered when possible and especially when one is sweeping. Some mold gives bread, cheese, and other food a bad taste, but it will not make one sick.

=How Germs Grow.=--Germs will not grow where it is very cold, but freezing the germs does not kill them. Boiling one minute kills most germs. Drying will stop the germs from growing, but will not kill all of them. Sunlight kills many of them.

Moisture and warmth make germs grow rapidly. A germ in growing lengthens out a little and then divides in the middle. It does this so quickly that one germ may become two in fifteen minutes. Each of these will then divide. In this way one germ can make many million germs in a single day (Fig. 18).

=The Spoiling of Meat.=--Fresh meat will not remain good even one day if left in a warm place. A large greenish blue fly seen buzzing about in warm weather will sometimes lay its eggs on meat. These will hatch the next day into little worms, called maggots. They grow rapidly and a few days later change into flies.

Germs will also spoil meat not kept cold. They feed on the meat and give off a poison, making it unfit to eat. The bad odor tells when the germs are at work. Every home should have a cold cellar or an ice box to keep food from spoiling.

=Saving Food from Souring.=--The souring of milk and of cooked food of any kind is due to the germs always present in the air and clinging by the thousands to unwashed dishes and hands. If meat or fruit is cooked and kept tightly covered, it will remain good for years. Many persons save fruit and vegetables for use in winter by putting them in jars, which are heated to kill the germs, and sealed tight to keep out other germs.

=Yeast or the Alcohol Plant.=--Sweet cider and other fruit juices are sometimes spoiled by a plant named yeast. This plant has the form of a football and is so small that a million of its kind together would not make a mass as large as the head of a pin. It floats about in the air and is present on the skins of fruits.

Yeast is also called the alcohol plant because whenever it grows in a sweet substance like fruit juice it changes part of it into a biting substance called alcohol. At the same time it gives off a gas. It is this gas which forms the bubbling or frothing in beer.

The millions of yeast plants in the yeast cake bought at the store, when put into the dough for bread, grow and form gas. This pushes the bits of dough apart and makes it light. The little alcohol formed is all driven off in the baking.

The alcohol which yeast forms by growing in sweet cider is in a few weeks changed to vinegar by other germs called the vinegar plants. Sour cider may make those who use it sick and drunk because it contains alcohol. Yeast makes wine out of grape juice.

PRACTICAL QUESTIONS

1. Where are germs found?

2. What is the form of microbes?

3. Name some diseases caused by germs.

4. What is mold?

5. Why should food be kept covered when not in use?

6. What causes meat to spoil?

7. How may fruit be kept from spoiling?

8. Where is yeast found?

9. What effect has yeast on fruit juice?

10. Why should you not drink sour cider?

CHAPTER VI

MILK MAY BE A FOOD OR A POISON

=Of what Milk is Made.=--Milk is the most perfect food known. It contains everything needed to build and strengthen the body. In one gallon of milk there is about one teacupful of pure fat, nearly the same amount of sugar, one teacupful of body-building food needed to make muscle and blood. There is also some lime and other mineral matter to make the bones of the young grow strong. The remaining seven pints are water.

=Kinds of Milk.=--When milk is left standing in a jar for several hours, much of the fat, which is present in the form of tiny balls, rises to the upper part. This upper layer of milk full of fat is called cream. If this is removed, the rest is called skim milk.

Milk after standing in a warm place one or two days becomes sour. It is then sometimes put into a tight box or barrel and beat in such a way as to break up the little balls of fat. These are then pressed together into a mass called butter. It requires a whole gallon of milk to make one teacupful of butter. The milk remaining after the butter is taken out is called buttermilk. Cheese is made from milk.

=Milk as a Food.=--Milk is a healthful drink for nearly every one and especially useful for those with weak bodies. During sickness it is sometimes the only food the patient can take. It is well for children to use two or three glasses of milk daily with their meals. It should be sipped slowly so it will mix with the fluid in the mouth and not form lumps called curds in the stomach.

A quart of milk contains more food for the body than a half pound of good beefsteak. A pint of milk will supply the body with about as much food as a pint of oysters. A bowl of milk and a half loaf of bread is a healthful supper for a boy or girl. Skim milk and buttermilk are healthful drinks which furnish much food for building bone, blood, and muscle.

=When Milk is a Poison.=--In New York, Cincinnati, and Chicago it has been noticed for many years that large numbers of babies become sick in warm weather and many of them die. The doctors learned that most of the babies taken sick were being fed on cows' milk because their own mothers did not have enough for them. It was then found that the sick babies had been using milk from dairies where the stables were dirty, the cows soiled, and the hands of the milkers unclean. On this account much dirt got into the milk.

Babies fed on clean milk from clean cows kept in clean stables remained strong and well. By much study the doctors learned that dirty milk is poisonous milk. The poison is made by the germs or bacteria living by the millions in unclean stables and in milk buckets not well washed in boiling water. Dirty milk becomes most poisonous in hot weather because warmth makes the germs grow very fast and become so numerous that millions are present in a teaspoonful of milk.

=Keeping Milk Clean.=--During one week of hot weather in Cincinnati, over a hundred babies were poisoned with dirty milk. In the same week twice this number were made sick by unclean milk in Philadelphia. During the hot part of the year in our country bad milk kills more than a half dozen babies every hour of the day and night.

The only way to have milk clean is to have clean stables with clean cows, milked by clean hands, and the milk handled in clean pails, cans, and bottles which have been scalded after being washed. The milk must then be kept cold until used, so that the germs will not grow in it.

=Saving the Baby from Bad Milk.=--If possible, milk should be bought for the baby in bottles sealed with a pasteboard lid. If milk turns sour the same day it is delivered, it is not fit for the baby to take. Heating it makes most milk safer for use. The heating of milk to kill most of the germs is pasteurizing it. It should be kept very hot for about fifteen minutes, but should not be allowed to boil. It should be cooled by placing the vessel on ice or in cold water.

The baby's bottle and nipple should be washed in cold water and then well scalded immediately after being used. The bottle, the nipple, and the milk should be kept away from flies and dust. One fly has been known to carry on its body more germs than there are leaves on a large tree.

=Flies and Fever in a Prison.=--In August, 1908, thirteen prisoners in the jail at Easton, Pennsylvania, were taken ill with typhoid fever. They had not been near any sick persons and their food and water were found to be pure. All those sick were in cells in one end of the prison. About twenty feet from this end a sewer had been uncovered two weeks before and left open. This sewer carried the waste from the hospital where several patients were sick with the fever. Flies fed on the waste in the sewer and then with the germs sticking to their feet flew into the cells of the prisoners and walked over their cups, spoons, and food. A little girl who played near this open sewer and shared her lunch with the flies had a severe attack of fever two weeks later because the germs scraped from the flies' feet on her food got into her body and grew.

=Milk and Disease.=--We must be very careful to get not only clean milk but milk from healthy cows milked by persons who have no typhoid fever, scarlet fever, or diphtheria in their homes. If only one or two disease germs get into the milk from the hands of those who have nursed the sick, these will grow into immense numbers in a single day. Many of those who use the milk will then become ill. Hundreds are made sick in this way every year.

PRACTICAL QUESTIONS

1. Why is milk a good food?

2. What does a gallon of milk contain?

3. What is cream?

4. How is butter made?

5. For whom is milk specially good?

6. How does milk become poisonous?

7. Why is dirty milk more poisonous in hot weather?

8. Tell what harm unclean milk does.

9. How may milk be kept clean?

10. Explain how milk is heated to make it safe for use.

11. Show how flies may cause fever.

12. Tell how milk may carry diphtheria into our homes.

CHAPTER VII

HOW THE BODY USES FOOD

=Organs for making ready the Food.=--Before the food can get into the blood and be carried over the body to feed the muscles and the brain, it must be made into a fluid. This changing of the solid food into a liquid by the stomach and other organs is called digestion. The organs which do this work are known as digestive organs. They consist of a food tube and several bodies called glands.

=The Food Tube.=--The food canal is about thirty feet long. Its first part, the mouth, opens back of the tongue into the throat, named the pharynx. This leads into a tube, the gullet, passing down through the back part of the chest into the stomach below the diaphragm. The stomach is a bent sac opening into a tube over twenty-five feet long called the bowels or intestines. This tube is folded into a bunch which fills a large part of the cavity of the abdomen.

=The Glands or Juice Makers.=--A gland is a little tube closed at one end, or a bunch of such tubes, which can take something out of the blood and make it into a juice. A gland under each ear and four others near the tongue make the juice called saliva which flows into the mouth through tubes.

A long, flat, pink gland back of the stomach is called the sweetbread or pancreas. This and a large brown gland, the liver, empty their juices into the intestines. The whole inner surface of the stomach and intestines is lined with tiny tubes, the glands. The juice of these with that of the other glands softens the food and makes it into a liquid.

=The Work of the Mouth.=--The mouth has three things to do: It should break the lumps of food into fine bits so it can be well wet with the slippery fluid called saliva and also easily swallowed. It must roll the food about so that it gets soaked with saliva. It must hold the food long enough to get much taste from it because this starts the juices to flowing into the stomach. Food gives out its taste only after it is changed to a liquid. It should not be washed down with water, as this weakens the juices in the stomach.

No food should be swallowed until it is broken into bits nearly as small as the head of a pin. Some foods, such as cheese, bananas, and nuts, should be made even finer than this. There is nothing in the stomach to crush to pieces large lumps of food. The juices of the stomach can do their full work only when the food is well chewed in the mouth.

=The Chewing of Food keeps away Sickness.=--Bread, meat, and potatoes should be cut into pieces no larger than half the size of your thumb and each piece put separately into your mouth with a fork. It should then be chewed from twenty to thirty times before another piece is put into the mouth. Food treated in this way will not cause headache or a sickness in the stomach called indigestion or dyspepsia. It is said that there are so many persons with this kind of sickness that more than $5,000,000 are spent every year for medicine to help them.

Too little chewing of the food while you are young may not cause many aches or pains, but if you form the habit of rapid eating it is hard to learn to eat slowly. No one who chews his food poorly can avoid sickness long or grow well and strong.

=The Work of the Stomach.=--When the food is swallowed, it passes through the gullet into the stomach. This is a sac holding more than a quart (Fig. 27). It is made of an outer wall of muscle and an inner skinlike coat full of tiny tubes called gastric glands. Millions of these give out drop by drop a watery fluid named gastric juice. This juice begins to flow as soon as we smell or taste food and continues to drop out as long as there is any food in the stomach.

The use of the gastric juice is to help change part of the food into a more watery fluid. To do this it must be well mixed with the food. This mixing is done by the muscles in the outer wall of the stomach (Fig. 29). They squeeze together and then loosen up in such a way as to move the food about and turn it over until every particle is wet again and again with the gastric juice.

=How long Food stays in the Stomach.=--A ring of muscle around the end of the stomach keeps the food from escaping until it has become a thin grayish liquid. The stomach can finish its work on some kinds of food in one or two hours. With other foods it must work four or five hours.

The stomach can finish its work on soft boiled eggs, milk, roasted potatoes, and broiled lamb within two hours. With pork, veal, cabbage, and fried potatoes it must work four or five hours. When a person is sick the stomach is weak, and he should have only the food which causes the stomach the least work.

=The Work of the Intestines.=--The last part of the work in getting the food ready for the blood is done in the long folded tube known as the intestine (Fig. 27). Here juices coming from the pancreas and liver mix with the food and change into a liquid those parts not acted on in the stomach.

The intestine does quite as much work as the stomach. Sometimes when the stomach is sick, too much work is put off on the intestines and then they become sick and give much pain.

The pint of watery fluid from the pancreas and the quart of greenish yellow fluid called bile given out by the liver are carried through two tubes into the intestine (Fig. 27). To mix these juices with the food the intestine is being swung gently back and forth and the walls squeezed together by muscles forming its outer coat. As soon as the intestine has finished its work the food begins to enter the blood.

=How Food gets into the Blood.=--An hour or two after food has entered the intestine it is almost as thin a fluid as milk. Millions of tiny fingerlike growths stick out from the inner side of the intestines and drink in the watery food. These little fingers for drinking up the food are scarcely one fourth as large as the point of a pencil. They are called villi.

The villi are filled with blood tubes having thin walls. The food passes through these walls into the blood stream. Much of it then goes to the liver, but the fatty parts flow up a tube along the backbone and empty into a blood tube in the neck. From the neck and the liver the food goes with the blood to the heart which sends it to all parts of the body.

=What the Liver does.=--The liver is a dark red body nearly as large as the upper half of your head. It lies just below the diaphragm. It works night and day helping to keep the inner parts of the body clean and at the same time deal out food.

The liver takes some waste out of the blood and sends it out into the intestine with the bile. When there is no food in the intestine, the bile is stored up in the gall bladder under the liver. The liver changes certain waste matter in the blood into such form that other organs can cast it out of the body. It also stores up certain parts of the food coming from the intestines and gives it out to the body little by little as it is needed.

=When and How much to Eat.=--When the food organs do not do their work rightly, the whole body becomes sick. Eating too much overworks the stomach. It becomes so full that the food cannot be moved about and well mixed with the juices. Germs then work on the food and make it sour. In fact the germs may change part of the food into a poison. This poison will cause headache and a bad feeling.

Do not form a habit of taking powders to cure headache. They are likely to hurt the heart. Take less food, eat it more slowly, and do not wash it down with drink. Stop eating before your stomach feels full.

Each meal gives the stomach about four hours of work to do. It then needs one hour of rest. This shows that the time from one meal to the next should be about five hours. Very young children and sick persons need food oftener. Boys and girls should not eat candies, cake, or other food between meals. It spoils the appetite and is likely to get the stomach out of working order.

=Danger Signals.=--A white or yellowish coat on the tongue, a bad breath, pain in the bowels, or a headache is a danger signal. It tells that the food organs are not doing their work as they should and unless help is given sickness is likely to occur. Medicine may help, but using foods easy to digest, eating less, chewing more, and getting plenty of exercise in the fresh air are likely to be the greatest aids to health.

=The Chewing of Tobacco and Digestion.=--Some men chew tobacco as much as ten hours every day. The taste of the tobacco makes the saliva flow from the glands into the mouth. This dissolves the poison out of the tobacco and it is then spit out. If the tobacco-soaked saliva were all swallowed, the man would be poisoned.

The chewing of tobacco causes the loss of much saliva which is needed to help digest the food. Anyone who tires his jaw by chewing tobacco is not likely to chew his food well. Some of the poison in the tobacco is taken into the body through the blood vessels in the lining of the mouth. This is shown by the fact that a boy not used to tobacco becomes very sick after he has chewed a mouthful for only ten minutes.

=Smoking and Digestion.=--Some persons think that the smoking of a cigar after a meal helps digestion. It may do so in some cases. If a lawyer is much excited about a case he is trying, or a business man is in trouble about his losses, the thinking causes the blood to flow to the head when it is needed in the stomach to give out digestive juices.

The taste of the tobacco smoke may cause some gastric juice to run out into the stomach, but at the same time it is likely to hurt the nerves of taste so that food cannot give so much enjoyment as when the nerves are unharmed. Although smoking may at the time help digestion a little, the poison in the tobacco may afterward injure the body. This poison is especially harmful to growing bodies, and boys who are wise will refuse to smoke on all occasions.

=Beer and Digestion.=--Some people drink beer with their meals because they think it makes the food taste better. It really prevents them from getting the full taste of the food because they wash it down before it is well soaked with the saliva.

The flavor of beer may sometimes cause an extra flow of gastric juice into the stomach, but the alcohol in the beer is likely to make the movements of the stomach slower. This prevents the food from being well and quickly mixed with the juices. Several glasses of beer used at one meal will make the stomach do its work very slowly, and it will not do it well.

=Wine and Digestion.=--Wine is taken by some people to give more appetite for food. It is likely, however, to do more harm than good because the alcohol in it makes the muscles which mix the food in the stomach act more slowly. Some of the food may sour before it gets wet with the juice. Much wine used at a meal is always harmful.

=Natural Appetite.=--If one is in health, he should feel a desire for his food at every meal. This desire for a reasonable amount of food is a natural appetite. Fresh air and exercise will do much to give one the right kind of an appetite. The eating of much sweets and the breathing of bad air are likely to spoil the appetite.

The use of some things, such as opium, tobacco, beer, wine, and whisky, creates an unnatural appetite. That is, after one has used these articles a few months he cannot stop their use without great suffering. The younger the person, the sooner the appetite becomes fixed. For this reason young persons should never use tobacco or alcoholic drinks of any kind.

PRACTICAL QUESTIONS

1. What is digestion?

2. Name the parts of the food tube.

3. Where does saliva come from?

4. Explain how the food is acted on in the mouth.

5. Why should food be well chewed?

6. What forms the gastric juice?

7. Of what use is the gastric juice?

8. How long does food stay in the stomach?

9. Name some foods easily digested.

10. What does the intestine do?

11. What are villi?

12. Tell how the food gets into the blood.

13. Of what use is the liver?

14. Why should we not eat too much?

15. Should we eat between meals?

16. Give three reasons why you should not use tobacco.

CHAPTER VIII

THE CARE OF THE MOUTH

=Sickness often begins in the Mouth.=--A clean mouth and sound teeth have much to do in keeping one well. The germs which cause nearly a half million deaths in the United States every year enter the body through the mouth. If the mouth is unclean, only one or two disease germs entering it may remain there and grow.

It is just as important to wash the mouth two or three times each day as it is to wash the hands and face. A few germs of diphtheria, sore throat, or tuberculosis are likely to get into the mouth any day, but if the mouth and teeth are well washed with a brush morning and night, the germs will not have time to grow and cause sickness.

=The Teeth.=--The first twenty teeth that appear are called the milk set. The eight front teeth grow out during the first year of life and back of these twelve others appear during the second year. Between the seventh and the tenth year all of the milk teeth are lost because others grow beneath them and push them out.

The first four teeth of the second set appear in the sixth year, just behind the last milk teeth (Fig. 30). These teeth should be watched very closely and at the first sign of decay you should go to the dentist. As the milk teeth get loose and come out, the second set of teeth take their places.

If you are ten or eleven years old, you should have twelve good teeth in the upper jaw and the same number below. The last ones to break through the gums are the four wisdom teeth at the back of the mouth. They appear after the seventeenth year.

The front teeth are called incisors because they are used to cut the food. The back teeth are named molars because they are used in grinding the food.

=Toothache.=--Toothache is a common ailment, and yet it can be entirely prevented. A tooth does not ache until it has a hole in it. The tender nerve within gives us warning that it is being hurt. The dentist can stop the ache and mend the tooth so that it will not ache again. Look at your teeth every month and feel about them with a wooden tooth-pick to know when the decay begins. If the little holes are mended as soon as found, you will never have toothache, and you can keep your teeth as long as you live.

=How to keep the Teeth Sound.=--Every tooth is covered with a layer of hard shining substance called enamel (Fig. 33). So long as this is unbroken the softer bony part of the tooth cannot decay. At the base of the tooth where the gum joins it the enamel is very thin, so that the scratch of a pin or other instrument may break it.

Never pick the teeth with a pin or needle. The biting off of thread, finger nails, and other hard material may crack the enamel. It may also be softened and eaten away by acid formed where food remains about a tooth. For this reason a quill or wooden pick or piece of tough thread, called dental floss, should be used to clear the teeth of food after each meal. Slimy matter collects over the whole surface of the teeth, and is likely to cause decay in spots unless it is cleaned off night and morning with brush and water. The chewing of dry crusts of bread or crackers strengthens the teeth and keeps off decay.

=Why Candy and other Sweets cause the Teeth to Decay.=--A sour substance called acid usually starts the decay of a tooth by eating through the enamel. Germs change sugar and other sweets into an acid. The acid is not made at once. An hour or more is needed for the germs to grow to form the acid. If, after eating sweet foods, the mouth is well cleaned, no acid will be formed. Sugar and candy do not, therefore, spoil the teeth unless it is left sticking about them.

=How to brush the Teeth.=--Every boy and girl should own a toothbrush. The teeth should be brushed every night and morning and kept white. Yellow or gray slimy teeth are very ugly. The teeth should be brushed on the inside as well as on the outside. It is best to brush the teeth crosswise for two minutes and then spend another two minutes brushing the upper teeth downwards and the lower teeth upwards. This prevents pushing the gum away from the teeth. Plenty of water should be used with the brush, and a little good powder is helpful once a day.

=How the Dentist can Help.=--Sometimes the milk teeth do not get loose so that they can be pulled with the fingers at the right time. The second teeth then come in at one side and may never get straight in place. They then spoil the appearance of the face and do poor work in chewing. The dentist should be asked to help straighten the teeth as soon as they appear crooked.

It is wise to have the dentist examine the teeth once or twice every year and remove a limy substance called tartar collecting at their base. The dentist can stop the decay in a tooth by cleaning out the little hole and filling it with gold or some other material. It may cause a little pain and expense to have the teeth filled, but it will save a hundred times as much pain and expense later. The six year molars need special care as they are likely to decay early. Even the milk teeth often need filling so that they will not be lost too soon.

=Bad Teeth cause Sickness.=--When anything decays, it is full of germs, and they are always giving off some poison. The poison may hurt the body and is likely to make parts of the mouth sore and tender so that other germs of disease can break through into the flesh. Disease germs can easily lodge in the holes of decaying teeth, grow in numbers, and finally cause diphtheria, sore throat, or other ailments.

Four out of every five children suffering from diphtheria or other throat or ear troubles are found to have from one to ten bad teeth. You must keep good teeth if you wish to be well and strong.

=The Value of Sound Teeth.=--Sound teeth which will do good work in chewing food are worth more than a foot or an arm. If the foot or arm is lost, the body is likely to get well and be as healthy as ever. The health of the whole body depends upon the work done by the teeth. Unless they do their part the stomach cannot get the food ready for the blood.

A part of badly chewed food is turned into a poison farther down in the food canal. This is what makes many people feel so tired and miserable much of the time. Hundreds of men have been refused admission to our army because they have poor teeth. Soldiers must be strong and well to take long marches and fight battles. Sound teeth give strength and health.

PRACTICAL QUESTIONS

1. Why should the mouth be washed out every day?

2. When do the milk teeth appear?

3. When are the milk teeth lost?

4. How many teeth have you?

5. How many show signs of decay?

6. How may toothache be prevented?

7. How may the teeth be kept sound?

8. Why do sweets cause the teeth to decay?

9. How should you brush your teeth?

10. Why should the dentist examine your teeth every year?

11. Why are sound teeth of great worth?

CHAPTER IX

ALCOHOLIC DRINKS

=Drink needed for Health.=--Water in the form of sweat and in other ways is constantly passing off from the body. This water carries with it the waste matter which, if it remained, would poison the body. There is some water in the food we eat, but not enough to supply the wants of the body.

Some persons think that the body needs beer or wine to keep it in good order. These liquids, as well as whisky, brandy, and rum, are called alcoholic drinks. The latest experiments and studies show that the body never needs alcoholic drinks to keep it in the best of health. These drinks sometimes make the body sick, and if much alcohol is taken at one time, the person becomes dizzy, staggers, and may fall down and go to sleep.

=The Desire for Drink.=--When parts of the body have too little water, there is a longing for drink. This is called thirst. As soon as a cup of water is drunk the desire is satisfied. There is no danger of drinking too much pure water.

Persons who have been accustomed to use alcoholic drink have a thirst which water does not satisfy. It is an unnatural thirst. Even beer or wine will not satisfy such a thirst except for a few minutes. Very often a person's thirst is not satisfied until he has used so much wine or whisky that he becomes dull and unsteady in his walk. He is then said to be drunk.

=How the Yeast Plant makes Alcohol.=--In the cake of yeast bought at the grocery there are millions of tiny plants, each shaped somewhat like a potato. This strange little plant will grow very rapidly when put into any sweet watery substance. It sends out a bud which grows larger and larger until in a half hour the bud is as large as the old plant. It may then break loose and grow other buds, just like the mother plant.

When yeast grows, it changes the sugar or sweet part of the water into alcohol and a gas called carbon dioxide. It is this gas which makes beer foam and bubble when opened. All alcohol used in beer, porter, ale, wine, brandy, rum, gin, and whisky is made by yeast plants.

In making beer, a sweet watery mixture is first prepared by mashing sprouted barley grains in water. Barley or any other grain forms sugar as soon as it begins to grow. Yeast plants are added to the sweet mixture. By growing they change some of the sugar into alcohol. Hops are also put in to give the beer a fine flavor. After a time the clear liquid is separated from the barley grains and hops and put into tight casks and bottles.

=The Making of Wine.=--Wine contains from two to four times as much alcohol as beer. Most of the wine is made in California, France, and Germany because grapes grow better in these countries than elsewhere. Wine may be made from the juice of any fruit, but the grape is generally used.

The grapes after being picked are thrown into large tubs and crushed so that the juice runs out. The wild yeast always present on the grape skins begins to grow in the juice and change some of the sugar into alcohol. This work of the yeast lasts from one to eight weeks. At the end of that time, the grape juice has become a kind of poor wine, consisting of alcohol, water, grape flavor, and some acid. To make the wine good it must be drawn off into casks, where the yeast causes further changes during several weeks. It is then put into bottles, where it should remain about five years to get the right flavor.

=Sherry= is a strong wine used in flavoring food, such as puddings and sauces. A few teaspoonfuls of this wine will make a child drunk. The wines made at home from elderberries, blackberries, and cherries contain alcohol which will do just as much harm as that in the purchased wines.

=How Brandy is Made.=--Brandy contains more alcohol than wine and almost as much as whisky. In fact brandy is only very strong wine. After the yeast plants have formed as much alcohol as they can in grape juice it becomes so strong that it kills them. This wine is then heated in such a way as to separate some of the water from it. The taking away of the water leaves the wine stronger in alcohol and it then forms brandy.

=Whisky and Rum.=--These two drinks are strong in alcohol. Nearly one half of each is pure alcohol. Whisky is usually made from rye, corn, or wheat, or all three together. They furnish the food in which the yeast grows and makes alcohol. This watery mixture of grain and alcohol is then heated and the vapor or steam forms whisky after it goes off through a pipe into another vessel. This kind of heating is distillation. Rum is formed in somewhat the same way from molasses or cane juice.

PRACTICAL QUESTIONS

1. Name some alcoholic drinks.

2. What is an unnatural thirst?

3. Explain how the yeast plant forms alcohol.

4. Tell how beer is made.

5. Tell how wine is made.

6. What is brandy?

7. Which drinks contain most alcohol?

CHAPTER X

ALCOHOL AND HEALTH

=The Money spent for Alcoholic Drinks.=--If the money spent for alcoholic drinks were all collected together in silver dollars, it would more than fill ten schoolrooms of average size. Not only rich men spend large sums yearly for fine wines and brandies, but also the poor give their money for beer and other drinks which the body does not need.

When parents waste their money on drink, they cannot buy the food and clothes needed to keep their families strong and well. In this way strong drink causes much sickness and suffering and sometimes even death.

=Alcohol injures the Body.=--Some persons drink very little beer or wine, so they seem to have but little effect on the health. Others use strong drink every day and for a few years they may remain quite well. Later ill health often comes on, and they then find that some of the organs have been so much hurt that they will never be quite well again.

A few years ago a group of fifty well-known men in the United States spent much time and thousands of dollars to learn how much alcohol was harming our country. After much study among many people they announced that there were about one million men and boys whose health had been injured by strong drink, such as beer, wine, and whisky. Because strong drink causes so much sorrow and sickness several states have passed laws forbidding its sale, and saloons have been closed by laws in parts of many other states.

=How Alcohol affects Kittens.=--The body of a kitten is made very much like the body of a child. It has just the same organs that a child has, and they do the same kind of work. Doctor Hodge, a well-known scientist of

Massachusetts, therefore concluded that alcohol would act on kittens in the same way as it would on a man or boy.

The doctor got two healthy kittens and fed them a little alcohol every day for nearly two weeks. In a few days they stopped being playful, did not grow, and did not keep their fur clean and smooth as healthy kittens do. After using alcohol several days they became very ill. This experiment showed that alcohol stops kittens from growing and robs them of good health.

=How Alcohol hurts Dogs.=--Doctor Hodge fed a little alcohol to two dogs nearly every day for three years. He also kept the brother and sister of these dogs, but gave them no alcohol. All the dogs had the same kind of food and were treated alike except that one pair got alcohol and the other pair did not.

The two drinking dogs got sick more easily and staid sick much longer than the temperance dogs. The drinking dogs became lazy, and timid, while the others were strong, full of fun, and brave.

Within four years the drinking dogs had born to them twenty-seven puppies, but only four of them lived to grow up. The others were too weak or sickly to live. During the same time the temperance dogs had forty-five puppies and forty-one of these lived. This shows that strong drink will not only injure the bodies of those who take it, but will make their children weak and sickly.

=The Use of Strong Drink causes Disease.=--Many persons who take beer or wine every day become fat. They think this is a sign of health. It is really a sign of disease. They become short of breath. They can no longer run so fast or do so much work because the heart is covered with fat and even some of its wall is changed to fat. For this reason the heart cannot do its work easily or well.

The kidneys which take the waste out of the blood often become injured by alcohol and a disease causing death follows. Sometimes the stomach becomes diseased so that it cannot do its work. This makes the whole body sick.

The hardening of parts of the liver is nearly always caused by the use of beer. The liver is sure to suffer if one uses much alcoholic drink because the alcohol goes direct from the food tube to the liver. Long use of strong drink may bring on disease in the brain and nerves.

=Alcoholic Drinks may cause Death.=--Every ten years the government appoints persons to visit each home in our land to take the census. A part of this census report consists of a table showing the disease of which people died. It is from the census report that we know that hundreds of people die every year from the use of alcohol.

=Danger to Health in beginning the Use of Strong Drink.=--A large number of people take a drink of beer or wine occasionally because they do not see that it hurts the body. No one expects to become a steady drinker or a drunkard when he begins to drink. Reports show that every drunkard begins his downward course by taking a few drinks occasionally. Thousands of persons begin a drunkard's life every year because the appetite leads them on gently until they become slaves and cannot let drink alone.

CHAPTER XI

TOBACCO AND OTHER DRUGS WHICH INJURE THE HEALTH

=How Tobacco is Made.=--Tobacco is made from the leaves of the tobacco plant. The plant may grow as tall as a man and bear more than a dozen leaves. Each leaf is two or three times as large as your hand. The seeds are planted in the springtime, and the plants are ready to be cut in the autumn. Most of our tobacco is raised in the Southern states and Cuba.

After cutting, the tobacco must be dried and cared for in a special way to give it the right flavor. It is then sent to factories and made into cigars, smoking tobacco, or chewing tobacco.

=How Tobacco is Used.=--Many million dollars are spent every year by the people of our country for tobacco. Most of the tobacco is used in smoking. Some men smoke it in pipes, while others smoke it in the form of cigars or cigarettes.

Many men chew tobacco. When used in this way, something like licorice is generally mixed with the tobacco to give it a more pleasant taste. Sometimes the dry tobacco is ground into a fine powder called snuff. This is used by both men and women.

=Tobacco contains a Poison.=--When boys chew or smoke tobacco for the first time, it always makes them sick. Chewing or smoking for fifteen minutes will make them grow dizzy and weak and feel so sick that they must lie down for a long time.

The sickness is caused by a poison called nicotine which is present in all tobacco. Much of this poison may be soaked out by boiling the tobacco in water. A cup of water in which a pipeful of tobacco has been boiled will kill goldfish in an hour when poured into a gallon jar of water with the fish. There is enough poison in a handful of tobacco to kill a boy who is not in the habit of using it.

=Why Men can use Tobacco without becoming Sick.=--Experiments upon animals have shown that the body can learn to use a poison and not become sick from it. The poison of a rattlesnake is deadly to most animals; but if a tiny bit of the poison is put under the skin of the rabbit one day and then on each succeeding day a little larger dose of the poison is given the rabbit for a long time, the animal will become so accustomed to the poison that the bite of a rattlesnake will not harm it. It is the same way with tobacco. Little by little the body learns to overcome the effects of the poison, but much use of tobacco is likely to hurt certain parts of the body.

=Tobacco is Harmful to the Young.=--A dose of poison which will kill a child may do but little harm to a man. Tobacco is certain to hurt boys more than it does men. The poison makes the body grow slower.

A large number of measurements made by Doctor Seaver showed that the boys who did not use tobacco gained in four years one twentieth more in weight and one fourth more in girth and height than the users of tobacco. These boys were between sixteen and twenty-two years of age. It is likely that tobacco will have a more harmful effect on younger boys.

=Laws to keep the Young Healthy.=--Boys ought to be wise and brave enough to let alone what keeps their bodies from growing and hurts their health, but some will not do it. For this reason some countries are trying to save the health of their boys by making laws against the use of tobacco.

The Germans a few years ago passed a law in their land forbidding all boys and girls under sixteen years of age to use tobacco in any form. Seeing the good results of this law in Germany and the harm that tobacco was doing the boys in the United States, the Emperor of Japan on the 6th of March, 1900, proclaimed this law: "The smoking of tobacco by minors under the age of twenty is prohibited."

In our own country several states have passed laws against the use of cigarettes by boys. One country after another is learning that if they want strong men, to fight, to work, and to win, tobacco must not be allowed to weaken the bodies of the young.

=How the White Man becomes a Slave.=--Before the Civil War the black men of the South were slaves. They could not do as they pleased because they belonged to their masters whom they must obey or else they would suffer punishment. No boy can begin the use of tobacco without the danger of becoming a slave to it.

The use of tobacco either by chewing or smoking gradually causes in any one the growth of an appetite which makes him feel miserable and unhappy unless it is kept satisfied. It can be satisfied only by the use of more and more tobacco.

Many men would like to quit the use of tobacco if they could do so without suffering. They are slaves, and tobacco is their master.

=Cigarettes and Health.=--A cigarette is a tube of paper filled with tobacco. The tobacco is usually not so strong as that used in cigars and pipes. For this reason, boys like it better, and because it is so mild they draw the smoke down into the lungs. This gives the poison a better chance to be taken up by the blood. On this account, and because one is likely to smoke oftener when he smokes a small piece of tobacco, cigarettes are thought by some to be more harmful than the use of tobacco in pipes and cigars.

=Tea and Coffee.=--Tea is made from the dried leaves of the tea plant. Tea plants are raised in North Carolina, China, and Japan. The drink called tea used at the table is made by pouring boiling water on the tea leaves. The leaves should not be boiled as this draws out a substance which keeps the stomach from doing its work in the right way.

Coffee is the seed of a plant growing in South America and Asia. It is roasted, then ground, and boiled in water to make the drink called coffee.

Children should not use either tea or coffee as they are likely to hurt the stomach and may injure the heart. One or two cups of tea or coffee daily seem to have little or no bad effect on the health of most grown persons. Coffee taken at supper may keep one awake by sending too much blood to the brain.

=Opium and Morphine.=--Opium is a dangerous drug which is got from the heads of the white poppy plant grown mostly in the far East. From gashes cut in the poppy heads a juice runs out and hardens into a gum from which the pure drug is made.

Some persons smoke opium for the drowsy and pleasant feeling it gives. Its use is very hurtful and ruins both body and mind. Morphine is a pure form of opium. Persons take it to kill pain and make them sleep. You should never take it except when given by the doctor, as a habit is quickly formed which will make you miserable through life.

=Patent Medicines.=--These are medicines advertised to cure ailments which generally cannot be cured by drugs. They are the medicines much advertised in the newspapers and magazines. Never use them unless your doctor tells you to do so. Many of them contain harmful drugs, such as morphine and alcohol. When you are sick, go to your doctor for advice.

PRACTICAL QUESTIONS

1. Explain how tobacco is raised.

2. How is tobacco used?

3. How does tobacco affect a boy using it for the first time?

4. What is the name of the poison in tobacco?

5. Tell how tobacco keeps boys from growing.

6. What countries do not allow boys to use tobacco?

7. What is meant by being a slave to tobacco?

8. What is tea?

9. What is coffee?

10. Why should you not use opium or morphine?

CHAPTER XII

THE SKIN AND BATHING

=Parts of the Skin.=--The skin is about as thick as the leather of your shoe. It is fastened to the muscles beneath with fine white threads like spider webs. This is called connective tissue because it connects the skin to the lean meat.

The skin is made of two layers (Fig. 45). The upper layer is formed of cells. This is named epidermis or scarfskin. The deeper layer is made largely of fine threads woven together. It is the true skin or derma. There is no blood in the scarfskin, but there is a network of blood tubes in the true skin. It is the crowding of these with blood that makes the skin look so red when we get hot or excited.

=The Use of the Skin.=--The skin has three chief uses. It protects the softer parts of the body from being hurt by rough or hard things which might touch it. It contains the organs of feeling. It helps keep the right amount of heat in the body.

The top part of the skin is dry and dead. This gives better protection than if it were moist and tender. Particles of it are wearing out and dropping off while other bits are growing beneath to take the place of the worn-out parts. The more this top skin is pressed on and rubbed, the thicker it becomes. For this reason it is twice as thick in the palms of the hand and on the soles of the feet.

Scattered through the true skin are millions of tiny organs fastened to the ends of the nerve threads leading to the spinal cord and brain. These organs tell us when the skin is touched or when it is hot or cold or is being hurt.

=The Pores and the Sweat Glands.=--On a warm day the skin becomes wet with a salty fluid called sweat or perspiration. This flows from the tiny holes or pores in the skin. A good magnifying glass will show these pores arranged in rows on the ridges in the palm of the hand.

From each pore a tube leads down into the true skin to a coiled tube forming the sweat gland (Fig. 45). Sweat glands are present by the thousands in the skin of all parts of the body. They give out from one pint to a gallon of sweat daily. The more we work and the warmer the weather, the more the sweat flows.

There is a little waste matter carried out of the body by the sweat, but its chief use is to cool the body. It does this by passing off in the air and carrying the heat with it. In this way the body is kept from getting too hot in summer.

=The Color of the Skin.=--In the African race the color of the skin is black, in the Chinese it is yellowish, while in our race it is nearly white. The different hues are due to a coloring matter called pigment. This lies in the deep part of the scarfskin. Going out in the wind and sun causes more pigment to collect, and we say we are tanned. If the pigment collects in spots, it makes freckles.

There is no way of removing at once freckles or tan. They usually disappear in the winter. No powders nor any other kind of medicine should be taken to make the skin white and smooth. Such medicines may contain poison and are likely in time to hurt the body. The skin may usually be kept soft and smooth by washing well with soft water and good soap. If it becomes harsh or cracked, a little glycerine rubbed on after each washing may help it.

=The Nails and their Care.=--The nails are hardened parts of the epidermis. They are intended to prevent the ends of the fingers from being hurt and to give a neat appearance to the hand.

The ends of the nails should never be chewed or torn off, as this makes the fingers blunt and the flesh sore. They should be filed or cut neatly with the scissors so that they do not stick out beyond the ends of the fingers.

Many boys and some girls spoil the appearance of their nails by letting a line of black dirt remain beneath them. A piece of a stick or a nail cleaner should be passed beneath the nails every time the hands are washed. If the fingers are much soiled, a stiff brush is useful in removing the dirt under the nails.

=The Hair.=--Some hair grows on nearly all parts of the body. It is much thicker on the head than elsewhere. Each hair grows from a little knob at the bottom of a tiny tube in the skin called the hair sac (Fig. 47). If hair is pulled out, another one will grow in its place if the knob at the bottom of the sac is not hurt.

One or two oil glands open into each hair sac and give out an oil to keep the scalp and hair soft. No other hair dressing is needed.

After thirty or forty years of age the hair begins to turn gray. No medicine will prevent the hair from turning gray, and it is generally unwise to color the hair with a dye. There is poison in some of the mixtures sold to color the hair.

=The Care of the Hair.=--When the hair is uncombed, the whole person looks untidy. The hair should be combed carefully every morning and again made tidy before each meal. You should use as little water as possible to moisten the hair. The glands can be made to give out their hair oil by squeezing parts of the scalp between the fingers.

The scalp should be well cleansed with soap and warm water every three or four weeks. The hair should be dried quickly with a soft towel and by sitting in the sun or near a stove. One is likely to catch cold by going out of doors when the hair is wet. Hair oils and dandruff cures should not be used unless advised by a physician. Pinching and wrinkling the scalp twice weekly with the fingers makes the blood tubes grow larger and bring more food to the hair. It will also in many persons stop the hair from falling out and prevent dandruff and itching.

Do not use the hair brush of another person or exchange hats with your companions. Unclean persons and those living or playing much with them often have among their hairs little creatures called head lice. They suck blood and cause constant itching. The doctor will tell any one how to get rid of them easily.

=Keeping the Skin Clean.=--The amount of dead matter carried out by the sweat on to the skin every day is equal to a mass as large as your thumb. Dust also works through the clothing and sticks fast to the moist skin. For this reason every one should wash the whole body once or twice each week. The feet should be washed oftener as they become more soiled.

Many persons take a bath every day. A cold bath taken just after rising in the morning wakes up the nerves, makes the heart work better, and gives health and strength to the whole body. Afterward, the body should be well rubbed with a coarse towel. The bath may be taken by lying in a tub of water or by rubbing the body over quickly with a wet sponge. A hot bath is best for cleansing the skin. A warm bath makes one sleepy and should, therefore, be taken only at bedtime.

The hands should always be well washed before handling food. Persons neglecting to do this have caused much sickness because of the disease germs on their hands. One hundred and fifty persons were given typhoid fever in one city in Massachusetts by a man who handled milk without washing his hands. Dirt and disease are companions. You must be clean if you would be healthy.

=The Kidneys.=--The sweat glands do not take out of the blood one quarter as much waste matter as the kidneys. These are two bodies longer than the finger and more than twice as wide, and having the shape of a bean. One lies on either side of the backbone below the liver.

The blood coming to the kidneys is full of waste and dead matter picked up from all parts of the body. This is passed out through the thin walls of the thousands of little blood tubes into the many tiny tubes of the kidneys.

Water is required to keep the body clean within as well as without. For this reason you should drink more than a quart of water daily. A glass or two of water drunk a half hour before meals cleanses and rouses to action the digestive organs.

=Alcohol and the Skin.=--The skin of those who use much beer or whisky often becomes rough, red, and pimply. Any alcoholic drink is likely to injure the skin because it may hinder good digestion. The drunkard has a red nose and a dark-colored skin. This is because alcohol weakens the walls of the blood tubes and lets them become gorged with blood.

If a person takes a drink only once in a while, his face becomes red after each drink, and an hour or two later the effect of the alcohol passes off. The blood tubes have squeezed up to their natural size.

=Alcohol and the Kidneys.=--Taking several glasses daily of even such weak alcoholic drink as beer often causes the kidneys to become sick. Some of their working parts become changed to fat and some parts become hard. The cells which let the waste matter pass out of the blood get hurt by the poison of the alcohol so that they let some of the food also pass out of the blood.

PRACTICAL QUESTIONS

1. Name the two parts of the skin.

2. Give the three uses of the skin.

3. What is a sweat gland?

4. How much sweat is formed daily?

5. Of what use is the sweat?

6. How should the nails be cared for?

7. Tell what care should be given the hair.

8. Why should you not use another person's hair brush?

9. Why should the skin be washed often?

10. Of what use is a cold bath?

11. Why should the hands be well washed before handling food?

12. Why does the drunkard have a red nose?

CHAPTER XIII

CLOTHING AND HOW TO USE IT

=Kinds of Clothing.=--People are beginning to learn that the wearing of the right kind of clothing has much to do with keeping them well. Many persons wear too heavy clothing in winter. Keeping the body too hot makes it weak.

Some kinds of clothing are much warmer than others. Some are expensive and others are cheap. Cheap clothes will often serve the same purpose as the more costly ones. If you look at your handkerchief or stockings, you will see that they are made of threads running crosswise to each other. All clothing is made from threads. Some of these are wool, some are linen, a few are silk, and many are cotton.

=Woolen Clothing.=--Woolen clothing, such as overcoats and fine cloth dresses and suits, is made from the wool cut from sheep. Enough wool can be sheared from two sheep in one year to make an entire suit of clothes. The raw wool is first twisted into threads and then woven by machines into cloth.

=Linen.=--Linen is used in making collars, cuffs, and handkerchiefs. It is made from fine threads taken from the flax plant. On a piece of ground as large as a schoolroom enough flax can be raised to make a half dozen collars. Garments to be worn in warm weather are sometimes made of linen.

=Silk.=--Silk is used in making neckties, gloves, ribbons, and dresses. Silk cloth is woven from the cocoons made by silkworms. A silkworm is about as big as your largest finger. It grows to this size from the egg in one month. In three or four days it spins a shell of silk thread completely surrounding itself. This shell is called a cocoon. Within this it changes to a moth.

When the cocoons are to be used for silk, the worm is killed by heat as soon as it has woven its home so that it may not change to a moth and eat off some of the silk in getting out. Many thousand worms are needed to get enough silk for a dress. The worms are raised largely in China, Japan, Italy, and France.

=Cotton.=--All calico, muslin, and most cheap clothing are made from cotton thread. This is made from the cotton fibers surrounding the seeds of the cotton plant (Fig. 52). The cotton used in this country is raised in the Southern states.

Cotton clothing is stronger and wears much longer than silk or wool, but it does not look so well and is not nearly so warm.

=The Use of Wraps and Overcoats.=--Outer wraps and overcoats should never be worn in a warm room or while working hard. They cause much sweat to form on the body, and as soon as one goes out of doors the sweat begins to pass off. This makes the body feel cold and in some cases leads to a long sickness.

When riding in cold weather, extra wraps should be worn. Scarfs and furs should not be worn about the throat except in extreme cold weather. Bundling up the neck and chin is likely to cause sore throat.

=Danger from Wet Clothing.=--Many children have caught severe colds leading to serious sickness by wearing wet or damp clothing. Wet clothing causes the heat to pass off from the body quickly, so that it is chilled before we know it. This may be shown by wrapping two bottles of warm water in cloths. Wet one cloth and let the other remain dry. In twenty minutes the bottle with the wet cloth will be cool, but the other one will still be warm. If your wet clothing cannot be changed at once, keep exercising or throw a heavy coat about you.

=Untidy and Soiled Clothing.=--All boys and girls should learn to keep their clothing as clean as possible. Do not wipe the hands on the clothing, or sit down in the dirt, or let food smear the front of the coat or dress.

The sweat is constantly bringing waste matter out of the body. This soils the clothing next to it. On this account clothing to be washed every week or oftener should be worn next to the skin. Very thin cotton underclothing should be worn in summer. Woolen clothes give more warmth for winter.

[Illustration: FIG. 53.--Showing how to prevent the shoe from pressing on corns caused by wearing tight shoes or socks roughly darned.]

=Shoes.=--Badly fitting shoes cause sore feet and much pain. A shoe that is tight across the toes is sure to cause corns. A corn is a thickened part of the top skin which presses on the more tender part beneath. Soaking the feet in hot water and filing off the top of the corn or using a corn plaster will help it. Shoes should always be a half inch longer than the foot. Waterproof shoes or rubbers should be worn in wet weather. Rubbers should not be worn in the house.

=Alcohol and Clothing.=--Many persons think that a drink of whisky will make them warm when taken on a cold day. For this reason whisky is sometimes used when clothing is really needed. The use of whisky or any other alcoholic drink will not make the body warm. It may make one feel warm because it loosens the muscles in the blood tubes of the skin and so lets more blood come to the surface. In this way the body becomes colder because too much blood gets into the skin and is then chilled by the cold air. As alcohol deadens the feeling it may prevent one from feeling cold when the body is really very cold. Too little clothing and too much alcohol have been known to cause men to freeze to death.

=Experience in using Alcohol to keep the Body Warm.=--Doctor Hayes, who went as physician with Doctor Kane to explore in the Arctic regions, said that he would never again take alcoholic drink with him on such a trip. He declared alcohol was of no use in helping men to keep warm. He found from actual experience that those who use alcohol cannot endure cold so well as other people.

Doctor Carpenter, a well-known physician, tells of a crew of sixty-six men who tried to stay in Hudson Bay all winter. They used some alcoholic drink. Only two of the party lived through the winter. Later another party of twenty-two men passed the winter in the same place. They used no strong drink at any time and as a consequence all but two of them were reported well and strong in the following spring.

CHAPTER XIV

BREATHING

=The Lungs.=--The lungs are two light spongy bodies filling up the greater part of the chest. The heart lies between the lungs. The lungs are formed largely of thousands of thin-walled sacs and two sets of tubes. One set of tubes carries air into and out of the lungs, and the other set is filled with blood. These sacs and tubes are held in place by a loose meshwork of tissue.

=Why we Breathe.=--Breathing means taking air into the lungs and forcing it out. The air is made to go into the lungs in order that a part of it called oxygen may get into the blood. The blood then carries the oxygen to all parts of the body where it can help the organs do their work.

The air which comes out of the lungs is not the same as that which goes in. Some of the oxygen has been used up and in its place is a heavier gas named carbon dioxide, which has been given out by the body. This carbon dioxide is part of the waste formed in every part of the body from the used-up food and dying parts of the body. We breathe therefore to get oxygen into the body and to take out some of the waste matter.

All animals must breathe. If our breath is shut off only four or five minutes, death results. In the earthworm the oxygen goes right through the skin into the blood. Bugs and flies have several little openings along the sides of the body which lead into tubes branching throughout the body to carry air. A fish gets air through its gills lying under a bony flap on each side of the head.

=How the Air passes into the Lungs.=--The outer openings of the nose are called nostrils. From here two channels lead back through the nose to the throat. The cavity of the throat behind the nose and tongue is the pharynx. At the bottom of the pharynx is a tube made mostly of gristle. This tube is larger than your thumb and is named the larynx, or voice box. The bump on its front part forms the lump in the throat called the Adam's Apple.

From the voice box extends the windpipe called trachea, down to the lungs. The windpipe divides at its lower end between the lungs into two branches.

One of these enters each lung.

=The Air Tubes in the Lungs.=--As the branch of the windpipe enters each lung it divides into smaller branches just like the limbs of a tree. These divide into still smaller tubes, which branch again and again until they are as small as a hair. These hairlike tubes have swollen ends called air sacs. The walls of the air sacs are much thinner than tissue paper.

=How the Blood trades Waste for Oxygen in the Lungs.=--The blood, which is constantly running from all parts of the body to the lungs, collects waste formed from the burnt food and dying parts of the organs. When the blood comes to the lungs, it is full of this waste, called carbon dioxide. The blood tubes divide into fine branches with very thin walls and form a rich network over the air sacs. This allows the carbon dioxide and water to pass out of the blood tubes into the air sacs, while the oxygen at the same time goes through into the blood. More than a pint of water is given off in the breath daily.

=How we Breathe.=--The bottom of the chest cavity is formed by an upward arching sheet of muscle called the diaphragm. This is fastened to the lower ribs. The ribs at rest slant downward and inward. When the ribs are pulled up or the arch of the diaphragm down, the cavity of the chest becomes larger. The air then runs into the lungs and swells them out. When the ribs are let drop or the arch of the diaphragm goes up, the air is pushed out of the lungs.

Without thinking, we work the muscles to draw up the ribs about eighteen times every minute, because all parts of the body are calling for oxygen. The harder we work the oftener we breathe because the muscles need more oxygen to make them go.

=Why we should breathe through the Nose.=--Most persons find it easy to breathe through the nose. In some, however, the passages in the nose are too small to carry the air without effort. On this account they let the mouth hang open and breathe through it.

The air should pass only through the nose because it is lined with hairs and tiny waving threads which catch the dust. In this way germs and dirt are prevented from getting into the throat and lungs, and in winter the cold air is warmed.

=Why Some Children cannot breathe through the Nose.=--When one has a cold, the lining of the nose becomes swollen and gives out a white substance called mucus. The swelling of the lining and the mucus fill up the passages. The nose should be kept clean by using a handkerchief and blowing out the mucus into it. Never put the finger into the nose. Disease germs often get on the fingers from things touched.

Children who have the habit of breathing through the mouth should be examined by a physician. He will, in most cases, find soft spongy growths called adenoids in the back part of the nose. They should always be removed as soon as possible. They may cause disease or deafness and may even injure the mind.

=The Voice.=--In the upper part of the voice box at the top of the windpipe is a fold of tissue stretched on either side. These two folds of tissue form the vocal cords. The air rushing past them causes sound. The different sounds are made by stretching the cords tight or loosely. By means of the tongue, teeth, and lips the sound is formed into words.

=How to use the Voice.=--A cold or much shouting makes the vocal cords swell and we become hoarse. Rest is the best cure. It is not polite to shout or whistle in the house and you should never use an angry tone of voice. When talking to a person, always speak distinctly but pleasantly and turn your face toward his and look directly into his eyes. Never use a harsh, loud tone of voice.

=Why you should not spit on Floors or Sidewalks.=--We used to think that any one well had no germs of sickness in his mouth, but we now know that many well persons have germs in their mouths which can cause long sickness when they get into other persons. If you are sick with diphtheria, scarlet fever, or sore throat, the germs of the disease are likely to remain in your mouth two or three months. Persons with tuberculosis throw out millions of these germs in their spit every day.

Spitting is not only an unclean habit but a deadly curse. Spit often contains the seeds of death. Women's skirts and the soles of our shoes carry it into the houses. It becomes dry, but the germs live and float about in the dust, then enter the mouth to make us sick. Carelessness with spit is said to cause more than a hundred deaths every day in our land.

=Do not use an Open Spittoon.=--It is much safer to have a smallpox patient in the house than an open spittoon in the summer. You can prevent the smallpox by vaccination, but you cannot keep the flies from carrying ten thousand germs of death from the spittoon to the food on the table. A million germs have been found on a single fly.

Spit should be dropped into a cup which should be kept covered when not being used. The spit should be destroyed by fire or some germ-killing fluid, such as lye or formalin.

=Keeping Sickness away from the Throat and Lungs.=--All sickness of the throat and lungs is caught from some one else. The germs are passed from one to another on the drinking cup, by sucking pencils, wetting the finger to turn the pages of a book, or putting the fingers in the nose or mouth.

Dust is the partner of disease. It contains germs. Avoid dust. Wipe up the rooms with a damp cloth; never use a feather duster. Avoid dry sweeping. Use a suction cleaner or have rugs which can be cleaned out of doors.

Give the lungs fresh air and deep breathing and the body good food and plenty of sleep to make it so strong that germs cannot overcome it when they enter.

=Alcoholic Drink and the Lungs.=--The most common disease of the lungs is tuberculosis. Nearly all bartenders who sell strong drink take some themselves. Lately it has been learned in Germany that tuberculosis causes one half of all the deaths among bartenders. Alcohol was once thought to be a good medicine for lung troubles, but it has been clearly proven that beer and whisky weaken the lungs and make them ready for the germs of disease. The body already weakened by the poison of the alcohol is then easily overcome by the disease.

=Tobacco and the Lungs.=--The occasional use of tobacco does not seem to hurt the lungs when fully grown. A study of many young persons has shown that the chest of smokers grows much more slowly than in those who do not use tobacco. As the lungs cannot grow any faster than the chest, they must grow slowly in boys using much tobacco.

Tobacco is a common cause of sore throat. Many smokers have been compelled to quit the habit because of throat troubles.

PRACTICAL QUESTIONS

1. Where are the lungs located?

2. What do the tubes in the lungs carry?

3. What part of the air do we use in the body?

4. Tell how the air gets into the lungs.

5. What passes from the blood into the air sacs?

6. Why should we breathe through the nose?

7. Why should you keep the fingers away from the nose?

8. What are the vocal cords?

9. Give two reasons why no one should spit on the floor.

10. Tell how alcohol harms the lungs.

CHAPTER XV

FRESH AIR AND HEALTH

=How much Air we Breathe.=--At every breath we take in about one pint of air. We breathe eighteen times each minute. Nine quarts of air therefore pass in and out of the lungs every minute. Air once breathed is not fit to breathe again. It contains waste and carbon dioxide which weaken the body.

If you breathe three full breaths into a wide-mouthed jar or bottle, it will contain so much of the carbon dioxide that a lighted candle or splinter will at once go out when thrust into the jar. A cat shut in a tight box two feet square and one foot high will die in less than a half hour.

Many years ago when the British and Hindoo soldiers were fighting each other, the Hindoos made prisoners of 146 of the British and locked them in a room about one half as large as a common schoolroom. There were only two small windows. During the night 123 of these men died because of the bad air.

=How much Air should enter a Room.=--The air laden with waste coming out of the lungs quickly mixes with the other air of the room. In this way all of the air in the room soon becomes impure. Forty children will give out nearly two barrels of air in one minute. In another minute this air has made all of the other air in the room unclean. It can still be breathed, but it makes children feel drowsy and lazy and may cause headache. They then do poor work.

To keep the air pure in a room, fresh air must be let in from the outside. If there are many in the room, the openings must be large or fans on a wheel must be used to force the air in. In the New York schools a little over a cubic yard of fresh air is forced into the room for each child every minute.

=How to get Fresh Air into a Room.=--When air is warmed it becomes lighter and rises. In many public buildings, fresh air heated by a furnace is forced into the rooms through pipes entering several feet above the floor. By a fan or heated flue the impure air is sucked out of the room through openings near the floor.

Changing the air in a room is called ventilation. To get plenty of fresh air in a room there must be one or more places for it to enter and one or more places for it to pass out. Where there is no furnace or fan, windows on one side of the room may be opened at the bottom to let in the air and the same windows opened at the top to let the impure air escape. Do not sit in a draft, but use a board or curtain to throw the air upward as it enters the window. A room should not be kept too warm. Sitting in a very warm room weakens the body and prepares it to take cold. The temperature of a living room should be between 65 and 70 degrees.

=Fresh Air while you Sleep.=--Thousands of people have weakened their bodies and brought on disease by sleeping in bad air. Many persons keep their windows so tightly closed during the night that the air smells bad in the morning. I knew a family who always slept with windows closed except in the very warmest weather. Three of the children died of tuberculosis, and a fourth one took the disease but was saved by keeping his windows wide open.

Bad air in the sleeping room makes one feel drowsy in the morning instead of refreshed by sleep. Your windows should always be open while you sleep. In cold weather a window should be open a foot at both the bottom and the top, or if there are two windows in the room, both may be opened at the bottom. In moderate weather the openings should be twice as large. A cap may be worn to keep the head warm, and the bed should be out of the draft.

=Fresh Air gives Health.=--Four hundred people die of tuberculosis in our country every day. A few years ago it was thought that no one could get well of this disease. Now three fourths of those in the first stages of the disease get well. The chief part of the cure is fresh air. Medicine is seldom used because no medicine will cure tuberculosis. Good food and rest are great helps.

Many of those with tuberculosis stay out of doors all day and at night sleep in tents or with all of the windows wide open, even in the coldest weather. Snow may blow in and the water in the room may turn to solid ice, but fresh air, the good angel of health, will give the body new strength and make it well and strong again.

Many years ago when the Indians lived in tents and often slept outdoors none of them had this dirty air disease of tuberculosis. Since they have formed the habit of living in houses nearly one half of some tribes have become sick with this catching disease.

=Making the Lungs Strong.=--It requires over three quarts of air to fill your lungs. When you breathe quietly, less than one pint of air passes in and out of your lungs. This shows that a large part of the lungs is not used. The air sacs at the top and in the bottom part of the lungs are seldom filled completely. It is in these places that disease begins.

Several minutes should be spent two or three times each day in exercising the lungs. Fill them completely with air many times. Learn to breathe deeply while you are walking in the fresh air. Hold the head up and the shoulders back so that every part of the lungs can be filled. Sit straight. Your life depends upon your lungs. Give them a chance to do their work and teach them to do it well.

=Tobacco and Pure Air.=--There is poison in the smoke of tobacco. This is shown by its effect on insects. Owners of greenhouses often buy the stems and other waste parts of tobacco. They pile it in a pan and after closing the doors and windows of the greenhouse tightly, set fire to it. The smoke rises and fills the whole house. In less than an hour it has killed many of the bugs and beetles which were destroying the plants.

A person not used to tobacco will sometimes be made sick by sitting only an hour in a room where persons are smoking. It is wrong for smokers to poison the air which others must breathe. For this reason a smoking room should be well ventilated.

CHAPTER XVI

THE BLOOD AND HOW IT FLOWS THROUGH THE BODY

=The Blood keeps the Body Clean within and gives it Food.=--Every tiny particle of the body, whether in the legs, arms, or head, must have food to keep it alive and help it do its work. It must also have oxygen, and it must be washed clean of its waste matter. All this is done by the streams of blood, which bathe every cell to bring it food and oxygen and to wash away its waste.

=Parts of the Blood.=--Blood consists of a clear, watery part called plasma and many little bodies named cells. The liquid found in a blister is the clear part of the blood. The cells which float in the watery part are so little and so close together that more than a million are in each drop of blood.

A few of the cells are white, but most of them are red, and it is their color that makes the blood look red. Your body contains about one gallon of blood. It is carried through the body in branching tubes called blood vessels (Fig. 70).

=The Blood Vessels.=--There are four kinds of blood vessels. They are the heart, the arteries, the capillaries, and the veins. The heart lies in the chest between the lungs. It squeezes the blood into the arteries. These carry the blood to all parts of the body. It then runs into the capillaries, which are tiny tubes connecting the arteries with the veins. The veins return the blood to the heart.

The blood flows so fast that it goes from the heart down to the toes and back again in a half minute.

=The Heart or Pump of Life.=--When the heart stops we die, because the blood can no longer flow to carry food and oxygen to the hungry tissues. The heart is a sac with thick walls of muscle. It is shaped like a strawberry and is about as large as your fist. Its cavity is divided into four parts. The two upper ones are called auricles and the lower ones are named ventricles. The blood enters the auricles and then pours through an opening into each ventricle, from which it passes out into the arteries.

=The Arteries or Sending Tubes.=--The blood is sent out from the heart through the arteries leading to all parts of the body. The chief artery is the aorta. It is larger than your thumb and extends from the heart down through the body in front of the backbone. It has more than twenty branches. All of these branch again and again like the limbs of a tree until they are finer than hairs.

A large tube, the lung artery, takes blood directly from the heart to the lungs. Here it branches into more than a thousand divisions, so that the blood can take in oxygen and give off to the lungs its waste.

=The Capillaries or Feeding Tubes.=--These are the tiny tubes, finer than hairs, which join the smallest end branches of the arteries with the beginnings of the little veins. They are so thickly scattered in the flesh that you cannot stick it with a pin without piercing one.

They are called feeding tubes because they have such very thin walls that the food in the blood and the oxygen brought from the lungs can pass through to feed the muscles and other organs. The dead parts of the body and also the ashes of the food used up, pass from the organs into the capillaries.

=The Veins or Returning Tubes.=--The veins, beginning in fine branches formed by the capillaries, return the blood to the heart. The branches unite into larger and larger vessels and finally flow into one main vein, the vena cava. This extends along in front of the backbone and opens into the heart.

=Why the Blood flows in only one Direction.=--The heart causes the flow of the blood. It does this by squeezing together its walls so as to make the blood go out into the arteries. When once in the arteries, the blood must go forward because there are little doors at the mouths of the arteries in the heart. These doors, called valves, open in only one direction, so that the blood cannot flow backward (Fig. 71). There are other valves between the upper and lower cavities of the heart, preventing the blood from being pushed back into the veins.

The movement of the walls of the heart in and out is called the heart beat. This can be plainly felt by placing the hand on the left side of the chest. The heart beats about seventy times each minute in grown persons, but much oftener in children. At each beat a wave of blood flows along the arteries. This is known as the pulse. It may be felt at the base of the thumb, where an artery runs just under the skin.

=Why the Heart sometimes beats Faster.=--When we run or do hard work, the heart may beat twice as fast as when we are lying down. This is because the muscles need more oxygen to help them act. Work makes them get hungry, and they send word by the nerves to the heart to hurry along the blood to bring more oxygen from the lungs.

When germs make the body sick, the heart often beats faster because it is affected by the poison made by the germs. The doctor then feels the pulse to tell how much the body is poisoned.

=Use of Blood Cells.=--The red cells act like boats. They load up with oxygen in the lungs and carry it to all parts of the body. Here they trade it off for carbon dioxide, a waste substance. This they carry back to the lungs to be cast out of the body.

There is one white blood cell to every four hundred red ones. The white cells are the body-guards. They change their shape and are able to crawl through the walls of the capillaries. Wherever the body is hurt, they collect in large numbers and eat the germs which are always trying to get into the body through sores. The white matter called pus in a sore is largely made of white blood cells which came there to fight the germs and were killed in the battle.

The germs of boils and fevers often get into the blood, but the white cells usually kill them before they have a chance to grow into large numbers and make the body sick.

=How to stop Bleeding.=--Most of the larger arteries are deep in the flesh and seldom get cut. There are many veins just under the skin. If the blood comes out in spurts, it is from an artery; but if it flows steadily, it is from a vein. If the blood does not run out in a stream, it will stop without any special care. As soon as the blood gets to the air it forms a jellylike mass called a clot. This helps stop the flow. All hurt places in the skin should be tied up in a clean cloth.

If a large artery is cut, a bandage twisted tight with a stick around the limb on the side of the wound next to the heart will stop the bleeding. If a vein is cut, the bandage should be placed on the side of the cut away from the heart.

=Alcoholic Drinks weaken the Blood.=--It has been noticed for some years that when a user of beer or whisky is attacked with fever, the disease is more severe than in one not using alcohol. The reason for this has lately been explained by a well-known scientist working in Paris. He put certain disease germs in rabbits, but they did not become sick. When he gave them a little alcohol and put the same amount of disease germs in them as before, they became sick and died. By careful study he learned that the white blood cells had in the first case killed the germs. In the second experiment the blood cells were made so weak and lazy by the alcohol that they did not put up such a strong fight against the germs.

=Tobacco and the Blood.=--Any one who chews or smokes tobacco regularly gets much of the poison into the blood. The vessels in the mouth and throat drink in some of the juice and also the poison from the smoke. How much this poison affects the blood cells is not known, but it is likely to do them some harm because it makes the growing cells of the body less active.

=How Beer weakens the Heart.=--Whisky was at one time thought to strengthen the heart, but doctors generally agree now that it weakens the heart. It may make the heart beat a little stronger for a few minutes, but after that the beating is weaker than usual.

Much use of beer is known to make fat collect around the heart and also cause some of the heart muscle itself to change into fat. In this way the heart becomes so weak that it can no longer do its work, and death results. The reports from Germany show that hundreds of persons die every year from weakened hearts made so by the use of much beer.

=Alcohol hurts the Blood Vessels.=--Careful examination of the blood vessels of drunkards after death shows that in many cases the alcohol has caused the walls of the vessels to become thick and sometimes hard. The thickening of the wall makes the channel of the tube smaller. The heart must then work much harder to get the blood through to feed the tissues.

=Tobacco and the Heart.=--Many boys who use tobacco regularly do not have a steady heart beat. This is specially true of those who smoke several cigarettes daily. A few years ago, when our country was at war with Spain, thousands of young men, wanted for soldiers, were examined to find out whether their bodies were strong enough to endure the hardships of war. Hundreds were refused admittance to the army because of weak bodies, and many of them were reported by the physicians as having hearts weakened by the use of tobacco.

The boys preparing for the army at the Military Academy at West Point and for sea fighting at the Naval Academy at Annapolis are not allowed to smoke cigarettes. Our country must have strong men for hard work. Tobacco never gives strength, but often causes weakness.

CHAPTER XVII

INSECTS AND HEALTH

=Malaria or Chills and Fever.=--Malaria is a disease in which the patient usually has a chill followed by a fever at the same time each day or every other day. Thousands of people suffer from this sickness in the warm parts of our country and hundreds of them die every year. In some regions people cannot live because this sickness attacks every one who comes there.

Many years ago a doctor found in the blood of malaria patients tiny animals. He thought that they might be the cause of the illness, but he could not find out how they got into the blood.

=Finding out how Malaria Germs get into the Blood.=--It had been noticed for many years that mosquitoes were always found wherever there was malaria. In the year 1900 two men decided to find out if they could live in a malaria region and not have the disease when the mosquitoes were kept from biting them.

They made their home a whole season in a cottage in the midst of many persons who were sick with malaria. They breathed the same air, ate the same kind of food, and drank the same kind of water as those who suffered from the disease, but they remained well. The only thing that they did different from those who got sick was to keep the mosquitoes out of their rooms at night by means of screens. This experiment and many other studies have shown that we catch malaria only by the bites of mosquitoes.

=Only a Few Mosquitoes carry Malaria.=--Malaria is not common in all regions where mosquitoes live, and it has been found that only one group of mosquitoes carries the germs. The two common groups are the straight-backed and the humped. To prove that the straight-backed ones did the harm several of them were allowed to suck blood from a man sick with malaria in Italy. They were then sent to London and let bite a healthy man. In a few days he became sick with malaria. Many experiments with the humped-back mosquitoes, found nearly everywhere in our country, show that they do not carry malaria germs.

=Yellow Fever.=--Until 1901 yellow fever was the scourge of many cities in the South. Thousands of persons lost their lives from it. Wherever the dread disease broke out in a city many persons would flee to the country because they thought that they could not breathe the air without getting the germs.

Some persons thought that mosquitoes might cause the disease, and in

1900 experiments were carried out in Cuba to learn whether mosquitoes really did carry yellow fever germs. Seven men made their home in a room well screened to keep out the mosquitoes. They used clothing which had been worn by others sick with the fever and even slept on pillows and blankets on which yellow fever victims had died. Many persons thought that these bedclothes were full of fever germs and that all the men would surely get the disease. Not one of them, however, got sick although they lived in the midst of these soiled materials for three weeks.

Seven other men were chosen for another experiment. A large room was prepared and made thoroughly clean. Only clean bedding and clean clothes were used. The men were given pure food and pure water, but into the room were let loose mosquitoes which had been sucking blood from a person sick with the fever. In a few days six of the seven men became sick with the fever and one of them died. From these experiments and other studies we now know that this dreadful fever is carried from the sick to the well only by the bites of mosquitoes.

=How Mosquitoes Live.=--Before we can get rid of any pests we must know where the eggs are hatched and the young pass their early life. The eggs of mosquitoes are laid on standing water. The water may be in an old tomato can, a rain barrel, a cistern, or a large pond. A day or two after the mother lays one or two hundred eggs, they hatch into dark, wriggling objects called wigglers. In from ten to twenty days later they change into flying mosquitoes. These habits of life show that the easiest time to kill them is when they are young.

=Getting rid of Mosquitoes.=--During warm weather mosquitoes cause the death of more than a thousand persons in the world every day besides making many others very sick. To get rid of mosquitoes is to prevent sickness and death. In one year yellow fever killed over five thousand people in New York and Philadelphia because the doctors did not know how to stop the disease from spreading.

When this fever broke out in New Orleans in 1905, less than five hundred persons died of it because the doctors had then learned that the disease is spread only by the yellow fever mosquito. They therefore began killing the mosquitoes. Kerosene was poured over all the ponds and stagnant pools of water which could not be drained. This kills the young mosquitoes because the oil gets into their breathing tube which they stick up to the surface of the water to get air. All rain barrels and tin cans were emptied and cisterns were tightly covered. Men, women, and children worked week days and Sundays killing mosquitoes because they knew that they were saving human life. The destroying fever was stopped.

=Flies cause much Sickness.=--Very few people are afraid of house flies because they do not bite. Although they are so small and seemingly harmless yet we know that they cause many more deaths every year than mad dogs, poisonous snakes, and all wild beasts.

Flies crawl around among slops, in spittoons, and in other unclean places. In this way they get thousands of germs of tuberculosis, typhoid fever, and cholera on their feet and then scatter them over our food as they crawl about on the table, in the grocery store, or among the milk cans. In our last war with Spain more than a thousand of our soldiers were made sick with fever carried to them by flies.

In Denver, Colorado, in 1908 fifty persons were made sick with the fever by flies which fed on the slops from a sick room and then crawled around in the milk cans from which those who became sick used milk.

=How to fight the Flies.=--House flies lay at one time about one hundred eggs in the dirt thrown out of horse stables, in garbage cans, or in any other unclean place. In a day or two the eggs hatch into little white worms which feed on the dirt. One or two weeks later the worms change to flies.

Flies may be kept out of houses by putting screens in the windows and doors or by darkening the rooms when they are not in use. The few which gain entrance may be caught in fly traps. All food in the store or the home should be kept covered. It is not safe to eat candy on which flies have wiped their feet or to drink the milk in which they have washed them.

The surest way to get rid of flies in any community is for all the people to work together and keep the entire neighborhood clean. No dead grass, weeds, or rags should be allowed to lie in the backyards or alleys. The cleanings from stables should be hauled away every week or stored in tightly covered boxes. Garbage cans must have close-fitting lids, so that there will be no place in which the young may hatch and grow.

=Other Insects which carry Disease.=--In certain parts of Africa, the sleeping sickness has made ruins of prosperous villages. Thousands of the natives are dying yearly from this disease. The germs are carried from one person to another by the bite of a fly.

Some fleas carry the germs of plague, which a few centuries ago swept across Asia and Europe destroying hundreds of lives daily. The plague is now common in India and was present in California in 1908 and 1910. The bedbug spreads several kinds of fevers in warm countries and may also be a carrier of leprosy and typhoid fever. These facts show that insects are dangerous and should be kept out of the home.

Any one troubled with these little pests in the house may learn how to get rid of them by writing to the Department of Agriculture, Washington, D.C.

CHAPTER XVIII

HOW THE BODY MOVES

=The Need of a Framework.=--The body needs a stiff framework made of bones for three purposes. One purpose is to give it shape, a second purpose is to help the body move, and a third one is to protect from injury some of the delicate organs, such as the heart and brain.

The bones are nowhere separate but are joined together with tough bands named ligaments. All the bones together form the skeleton.

All animals from fish to man have a skeleton. Many of the lower creatures, such as worms and flies, have no bony skeleton. Most of these move sluggishly or have a hardened outer covering, like beetles and wasps. The skeleton of animals such as the cat, rabbit, or cow, has about the same number of bones as man, and they are arranged in the same way.

=Of what a Bone is Made.=--Although the bones are so hard, they are not dead. They contain blood, have feeling, and are just as much alive as the softer parts of the body. It is the lime that makes them stiff. This can be eaten out by putting the bone in strong vinegar or other acid for a few days. A long bone will then become so limber that it can be tied into a knot.

The living part of a bone can be burned out by placing it on hot coals for a half hour. At the end of this time the bone will look just as before, but when it is touched, will crumble to pieces.

=Forms of Bones.=--The bones of the legs and arms are hollow. This form gives the greatest strength with the least weight. You can prove this by using two sheets of paper. Roll one sheet and fold the other one. Hang weights on both ends of each and use the finger for a support in the middle.

The cavity of these bones is filled with a soft white substance called marrow. This is largely fat. Each bone is surrounded by a tough membrane to which the muscles are attached.

=Arrangement of the Bones.=--The bones of the head form the skull. The other bones of the body not belonging to the limbs make up the trunk. There are over two hundred bones in the entire body. Eight of these form a case for the brain. Fourteen give shape to the face. A chain of twenty-six bones named vertebr?forms the backbone.

Twelve pairs of ribs encircle the chest. They are fastened behind to the backbone. The front parts of the ribs are made of pieces of gristle. The seven upper pairs are joined to the breastbone. The five lower pairs are named false ribs.

The collar bone is in front of the shoulder and behind it is the flat shoulder blade. There is one bone in the upper part of each arm and leg and two bones in the lower part of each limb. Twenty-eight small bones are found in the hand, while twenty-seven are present in the foot.

=How the Bones may be Injured.=--In the young some of the entire bones and parts of many others are soft like gristle. For this reason, the bones of the young seldom get broken, but they are easily bent and pressed out of their natural shape. On this account you should hold the body erect in sitting and walking. Bending over the table or desk day after day is not only likely to cause round shoulders, but is sure to squeeze up the lungs and other organs so they cannot do their best work.

Sitting at a table or desk, so that one shoulder is higher than the other or carrying books at the side, so that they rest on the hip may cause a curve sidewise in the backbone. Tight clothing about the waist presses the ribs out of shape and hurts the other organs within the body.

=Caring for Broken Bones.=--When a bone of the arm or leg is broken, the muscles tend to make the ends shove over each other. The broken ends are sometimes sharp, and if the limb is bent, these may tear through the flesh. This may be prevented by binding a board firmly on opposite sides of the limb across the broken part. This will hold the bones in place until the surgeon comes and will also allow the patient to be moved.

The surgeon will set the broken bones by bringing the ends together and holding them in place by sheets of wood or metal firmly held by a bandage. In a few days the membrane around the bone begins to grow new bone to join the broken parts.

=How the Bones are joined together.=--The two general classes of joints are the movable and immovable. Except the lower jaw, the bones of the skull are so tightly joined together that there is no motion between them. The bones of the wrist and back have but little movement. The freest motion is at the shoulder joint, where the round head of one bone fits into the shallow cup of another. This is called a ball and socket joint. Such a joint is found also at the hip. At the elbow and knee the bones move back and forth like a hinge and these are named hinge joints.

=Working Parts of a Joint.=--The ends of the bones are covered with a thin layer of gristle. The bones are held in place by several strong bands called ligaments (Fig. 82). These entirely surround the joint. On their inner sides is a delicate membrane which gives out a slippery fluid to make the joint work easily.

The ligaments are sometimes strained, stretched, or torn by a fall. The joint then swells because the watery part of the blood collects there. A sprained limb should be elevated to prevent swelling. Bathing it in very hot water is helpful.

=The Muscles.=--The muscles form the lean meat in any animal. They make up about one half the weight of the body. Each muscle is a bundle of thousands of little threads held together by other finer threads, while the whole is surrounded by a thin sheet. Little bundles formed of several of these threads called fibers may be seen in a piece of cooked beef picked to pieces. There are over five hundred muscles in the body.

[Illustration: FIG. 83.--Fifty of the muscles just under the skin. Note the white cords, the tendons in the regions of the hands and feet.]

[Illustration: FIG. 84.--The biceps muscle contracted above and relaxed or loosened below.]

Some of the muscles are more than a foot long and have the shape of a ribbon. Some are circular like those around the mouth, eyes, and stomach, while others are large in the middle and taper toward the ends.

=How the Muscles are fastened to the Bones.=--The two ends of a muscle are attached to different bones. In many cases the muscle is not joined directly to the bone, but is connected to a tough white cord called a tendon. The tendon is then fixed to the bone.

Several of the muscles in the forearm run into tendons in the wrist because if the muscle part were to extend along the wrist, this part of the arm would be large and clumsy instead of graceful and slender. Some of these tendons may be seen to move by bending the wrist and then working the fingers.

=How the Muscles do their Work.=--A tiny nerve thread runs from the spinal cord or brain to every muscle thread. Messages sent through the nerve threads to the muscles make them act. A muscle can act in only two ways (Fig. 84). It can become shorter or longer. When it gets shorter, we say it contracts. When it stretches out, it is said to relax.

A muscle cannot contract more than one fourth of its length. To pull the forearm up, the brain sends a message to the muscle fixed by one end at the shoulder and by the other end to a bone at the elbow. The muscle at once becomes shorter and thicker, as may be felt by placing the fingers on it. Although it shortens only two inches it is fastened to the bone so near the elbow that it draws the hand up two feet.

PRACTICAL QUESTIONS

1. Of what use are the bones?

2. What animals have bony skeletons?

3. What can you say of the form of bones?

4. How many bones in the body?

5. Name six bones.

6. What part of the arm has two bones side by side?

7. How many ribs have you?

8. Explain how a broken bone should be cared for.

9. Point out and name two kinds of joints.

10. What are ligaments?

11. Of what is a muscle made?

12. How many muscles in the body?

13. How many tendons can you feel in your wrist?

CHAPTER XIX

THE MUSCLES AND HEALTH

=Making the Muscles Strong.=--No persons use all of the five hundred muscles in the body every day. In slow walking only about twenty muscles are used, while in running more than four times that number are called into action. Muscles which are not used get lazy and weak.

Every time a muscle is made to act the blood vessels enlarge and bring to it more blood to supply food. The more food the muscle has the stronger it grows. The right arm is used more than the left in most persons. This makes it so much stronger that some boys can lift twenty-five pounds more with the right arm than they can with the left.

=Using the Muscles keeps the Body Well.=--All muscles must have more blood when they are used so that the heart is made to beat faster and stronger by exercise. In this way its valves and walls become able to do more work. Such a heart not only does its work better in a well person, but is able to keep pumping when the body is weakened by disease. Many persons die because the heart gets too weak to push the blood through the body.

In all the little spaces between the muscles and parts of other organs is some watery part of the blood containing much waste given off from the tissues. Moving the muscles presses on this watery waste in such a way as to move it along into the blood channels. It then can be cast out of the body by the lungs and other organs. One reason why we feel so good after exercise is because the poisonous waste has been taken away.

No one can remain well very long without taking exercise. Children as well as older persons should enjoy one or two hours of outdoor play every day.

=How to exercise the Muscles.=--Outdoor games give the best form of exercise. Tennis, baseball, cricket, rowing, and swimming are sports which bring nearly all the muscles into use. Every boy and girl should learn to swim. It is dangerous to go swimming alone or to swim in deep water. Cramp may seize the muscles at any time, so that the limbs cannot be moved. Hundreds of persons are drowned every year by venturing in deep water.

Taking care of the yard and garden and helping with other work about the home is one of the best ways of getting exercise and at the same time doing some good.

=Special Kinds of Exercise.=--A room with ropes, swings, and machines in it for exercise is called a gymnasium. Under the direction of a teacher the pupils can get quickly just the right kind of exercise to strengthen the weak parts of the body and keep every organ in health. The muscles oftenest neglected are those of the chest. Every one should keep his chest full and round by swinging the arms and practicing deep breathing every day.

=Danger from too much Exercise.=--Lately it has been learned that very violent exercise for more than a few minutes often injures the heart. The running of many races until you are all out of breath or much jumping of the rope is likely to strain the heart. It is always harmful to urge the body on until it is completely tired out.

=Alcohol makes the Muscles Weak.=--In the year 1903 two learned men in Switzerland spent much time to determine whether alcohol helped persons do more work. They tried more than two hundred experiments with men to whom they sometimes gave wine and sometimes food, and sometimes both were given together.

The results of these tests showed that when wine was given alone, the man's ability to do work was increased for a short time, but later he could not do so much work as when he had taken no wine. When the man took both food and wine, he could do only about nine tenths as much work as when he took food alone.

The most careful tests by other persons show that whisky will not help a man do more work, lift a heavier weight, or shoot straighter. In fact little or much whisky makes him less able to do any of these things.

=Beer makes the Muscles Lazy.=--Doctor Parkes of Netley secured two gangs of soldiers to do the same kind of work. He allowed the first gang to drink some beer, but the second gang were not allowed to have any. During the first hour the beer gang did the most work, but after that the temperance gang did far more work during the entire day. The next week beer was refused the first gang and given to the second. The beer helped the second gang do more work than the first one for nearly two hours, but after that they did much less than the first gang. This shows that men who wish to do their best work during the entire day should not use beer.

=Tobacco and the Muscles.=--Many experiments and studies have shown that the body cannot do its best work when even very small amounts of poison are taken day after day. The poison in tobacco is believed to weaken the muscles so much that no man on a football team in any of our large colleges or universities is allowed to smoke or chew during the season. Persons training for any contest where much strength is required do not use tobacco in any form.

=Tobacco prevents Growth of the Muscles.=--The moderate use of tobacco by men has but little effect on the muscles. It may cause them to tire a little more easily when doing very hard work. Tobacco poison does, however, show a marked effect on the muscles of the young.

Very careful measurements made at one of the large universities showed that the boys who did not smoke grew one tenth more in weight and one fourth more in height than those using tobacco regularly. This slow growth in tobacco users is partly due to the fact that tobacco makes the muscles in the walls of the blood vessels squeeze together so as to shut off some of the blood from the legs, arms, and other parts, so that they get too little food. Tobacco may also cause less food to be digested for the use of the body.

CHAPTER XX

HOW THE BODY IS GOVERNED

=Making the Parts of the Body Work.=--Each of the hundreds of organs in the body has a certain work to do and this must be done at the right time. In order that all may work together and each one do its part when needed, there is a chief manager called the brain and a helping manager named the spinal cord. Millions of tiny threads for sending messages connect the two managers with every part of the body. These threads form the nerves.

=The Brain.=--The brain is a soft bunch of matter filling the inside of the skull. The bones of the skull are a quarter of an inch thick and prevent any common knocks from hurting the brain. It is surrounded by three coverings which also help shield it from injury.

The surface of the brain is very uneven. There are a great many folds separated by grooves. Some of these are more than an inch deep.

=Parts of the Brain.=--The brain is divided into three chief parts. The upper and larger part is called the big brain or cerebrum. The lower part behind is the little brain or cerebellum. The part under the little brain and round like the thumb is the stem of the brain. It connects the larger parts of the brain with the spinal cord.

The big brain is partly separated into halves by a deep cut called a fissure. Each half is a hemisphere.

The outer layer of the brain is gray. It is made of millions of tiny lumps of matter which are the bodies of nerve cells. These are connected by threads much finer than hairs with other parts of the brain and spinal cord. Over these threads called nerve fibers one cell can talk to another somewhat as we talk over a telephone wire.

=The Spinal Cord.=--This is a bundle of nerve matter about as thick as your finger. It extends from the stem of the brain down the canal in the backbone. The outer layer of the spinal cord is white because it is made of the tiny threads, nerve fibers. The inner part is made of the bodies of nerve cells and therefore looks gray. The fibers are branching threads from the cells in the cord and brain.

=The Message Carriers or Nerve Fibers.=--In order that the managers may send messages, these fine threads, the nerve fibers, extend from them to all parts of the body. In many places from five to five hundred or more of these fibers are united in one white cord called a nerve.

Twelve pairs of nerves are joined to the under side of the brain and thirty-one pairs are connected with the spinal cord (Fig. 86). The nerves of the brain branch to all parts of the head and neck, and one pair goes down to the lungs, heart, and stomach. The nerves connected with the spinal cord branch to every part of the muscles, bones, and skin of the arms, trunk, and legs.

=How the Nerves do their Work.=--On a telephone wire we can send a message in either direction. A message can travel on a nerve in only one direction. For this reason there must be two kinds of nerves. One kind is called sending nerves because the brain and cord send orders over them to make the organs act. The other kind carries messages to the brain from the eyes, ears, skin, or other organs of sense, telling it how they feel. On this account these are named receiving nerves.

When we wish to catch a ball, the brain sends an order along the nerve threads down the spinal cord and out through the nerves of the arm to the fingers to get ready to seize a ball. The fingers are spread to grasp the ball, but they do not close until a message goes from the skin of the finger tips to the spinal cord, telling it that the ball is in the hand.

=The Work of the Brain.=--The brain is not only the chief manager of the body, but the home of the mind. The mind acts through the brain. The mind receives through the brain what the eye sees, the ear hears, the nose smells, and the fingers feel. All this knowledge is stored up in the mind and called memory. These facts and others learned later are worked over by the mind. This is called thought.

The mind rules and becomes good or bad according to whether it contains good thoughts or bad thoughts. It is wrong to read books and papers about robberies and murders or to tell or to listen to bad stories, because in this way evil thoughts get into the mind. The best way of keeping badness out of the mind is to fill it with goodness. It is said that Lincoln was so busy thinking how he could help others that there was no room in his mind for a bad thought. Doing some kindness every day helps much in the making of a good mind.

=Habit.=--The doing of anything over and over again until the body goes through the same motions without any or very little thought is called habit. The brain and nerves are so formed that when they get used to obeying the same order of the mind again and again, they will carry out these orders when the mind no longer gives them. Sometimes they will continue to obey the old orders even when new ones are given.

Many persons would like to break off the habit of drinking beer or whisky, of chewing tobacco, and using bad language, but they find it very hard to make the mind rule the body because they have let the nerves have their own way so long.

Speaking cheerfully to those we meet, giving a kind word to our friends, and looking pleasant are good habits which every one ought to form in youth. They not only make the mind better, but they help the body to keep well and will prepare the way for success in life later. Nobody wants a grumbling clerk or a sour-faced housekeeper.

[Illustration: FIG. 88.--The difference in appearance between a pouting and a pleasant expression.]

=Parts of the Body work without Orders from the Brain.=--A snake with its brain crushed will still squirm and a chicken with its head cut off jumps about. These movements are caused by orders sent from the spinal cord. When the hand or foot is being hurt, the spinal cord orders the muscles to draw the limb away even before we feel the pain in the brain. Many of the movements of the body which are often repeated may be directed by the spinal cord, while the brain is left free to do other work. This is why the spinal cord is called the helping manager.

The action of the muscles in the walls of the blood vessels, the working of the stomach, the liver, pancreas, and other glands are not directed by the brain, but by the sympathetic nerves. These extend from a little cord on either side of the backbone to all parts of the body and make the organs, such as the heart and sweat glands, which we cannot make obey our will, do their work.

=Injury to the Nerves.=--The nerves are so important for the welfare of the body that all the chief ones are placed deep in the flesh, where they are not likely to be hurt. If the nerves leading to the arm were cut, it could not be moved, and we should have no feeling in it. The hurting of a part of the brain, the spinal cord, or the nerves may cause loss of feeling or motion in the leg, arm, or other part of the body. Such a part then seems asleep or dead and is said to have paralysis.

Pressing on a nerve prevents it from acting. Sitting so as to press on the nerve of the leg often makes the foot go to sleep. The bursting of a blood vessel in the brain may let a blood clot form and press on the nerves which govern the arm or the leg. This pressure may cause paralysis.

=Resting the Brain.=--When there is no food in the stomach, it has time to rest. When we sit down or lie down, the muscles get rest. The brain is always busy except when we are asleep. No one can live even a week without sleep. If a dog is kept awake five days, it will die.

Children need much more sleep than older persons. Men and women who work should have about eight hours of sleep daily to remain in good health. Children of twelve years should sleep nine hours each day; those of ten years, ten hours; those of seven years, eleven hours; and those of four years, twelve hours.

=Getting the most out of Sleep.=--You should go to bed every night at about the same hour. This will help you to fall asleep as soon as you are in bed. Do not sleep in the clothes which you have worn during the day, but hang them up to air, and put on a night robe.

Children should use a very low pillow, so that the body can lie straight in the bed. This gives the lungs and heart freedom to act. Do not lie on the back as this causes some of the organs to press on certain nerves and makes you dream. The windows should be opened wide because fresh air is the best aid to rest and health and keeps away tuberculosis.

PRACTICAL QUESTIONS

1. What makes the parts of the body work together?

2. Describe the surface of the brain.

3. Name the three parts of the brain.

4. Of what is the outer layer of the brain made?

5. Where is the spinal cord?

6. What are nerve fibers?

7. What work does the brain do?

8. What makes the mind good or bad?

9. What is habit?

10. How long should children sleep?

11. How can you get the most good out of sleep?

CHAPTER XXI

HOW NARCOTICS AND STIMULANTS AFFECT THE BRAIN AND NERVES

=What Narcotics and Stimulants Are.=--A narcotic is something which when taken into the body makes the organs do their work more slowly and tends to cause sleepiness. Alcoholic drinks, tobacco, opium, soothing sirups, and pain killers are narcotics.

A stimulant is a substance which makes the organs of the body do more and quicker work and does not later make the organs work more slowly. Coffee and tea are stimulants. Beer, wine, and whisky were once thought to be stimulants, but experiments have shown them to be narcotics. They urge the brain to faster work for a few minutes, but a half hour later they make it act slower than usual.

=Alcohol hurts the Brain.=--Within five minutes after a drink of beer or whisky has been swallowed, part of the alcohol has reached the blood. Within fifteen minutes much of the alcohol has gone from the stomach directly into the blood. In a minute after entering the blood vessels it reaches the brain.

If much strong drink is taken, the cells of the brain become so numbed that they cannot give the right orders to the muscles to move the limbs. The person then staggers about and is said to be drunk. Much whisky taken will make the nerve cells so numb that a man cannot move, and he will then lie down as if in a deep sleep.

A tablespoonful of whisky will make a child drunk and twice that amount may make him very sick. Much use of strong drink sometimes gives to the brain a terrible disease called delirium tremens. In this sickness the man thinks he sees horned animals, hissing snakes, and other creatures which annoy him.

=Alcohol injures the Thinking Part of the Brain.=--It was once thought that wine or whisky would make a man think better. Now we know that either of these drinks makes his thoughts slower and also causes him to make mistakes.

Two doctors in Europe made many tests with men to learn how alcohol affected their thinking. They found that when using wine the men could do about one tenth less work in adding numbers than when they took no strong drink. These doctors also tested the effect of alcohol on memory and discovered that the use of even small quantities of liquor caused their pupils to learn their lessons more slowly.

When persons have taken only a very little drink, they often say and do very foolish things. They sometimes tell secrets, for which they are very sorry when they get sober. Often they become angry at the least cause and strike or even shoot any person who seems to speak or work against them in any way.

=Alcohol makes People Steal and Kill.=--The alcohol in strong drink, when often used, appears to deaden that part of the brain which helps the mind know right from wrong. In one year the courts of Suffolk County in Massachusetts found 17,000 persons guilty of doing some wickedness and in over 12,000 of these cases alcohol was found to be the cause of doing the wrong for which they were arrested.

Some time ago there were collected the records of 30,000 prisoners, and among these over 12,000 had done their wicked acts while alcohol was numbing the brain. Lately another careful record of over 13,000 prisoners in twelve different states has been studied. In over 4000 of these men the use of strong drink was the first cause of their crimes.

=Alcohol makes the Mind Sick.=--Since the mind depends upon certain parts of the brain, whatever hurts the brain is quite sure to hurt the mind. When the mind cannot reason rightly, the person is said to be insane. A study of 2000 insane men in New York State showed that the use of alcoholic drink was the cause of the mind sickness in over 500 of them. Of 687 persons in Massachusetts who were so insane that they had to be cared for daily by others, more than 200 of them were brought to this sad condition by alcohol.

=Brain of the Young easily overcome by Alcohol.=--No one expects to become a drunkard or a criminal when he first begins to drink. The continued use of alcohol, however, soon numbs the brain and weakens the mind, so that the person's will power is lost. He is then not able to quit drinking even though he wants to stop. He has become a slave to alcohol.

The brain of a young person is injured much more quickly by alcohol than that of an older person and he is much more likely to become a slave than one who begins the use of drink late in life. Doctor Lambert, of New York, studied the cases of 259 slaves to alcohol. He learned that four began to drink before six years of age; thirteen between six and twelve years of age; sixty, between twelve and sixteen years; 102 between sixteen and twenty-one years; seventy-one, between twenty-one and thirty years; and only eight after thirty years of age. These facts teach that it is dangerous for the young to take strong drink at any time.

=Laws against Alcohol.=--The men who make laws for the good of the people are learning that alcohol is injuring the mind and body of many persons every year. For this reason laws have lately been passed forbidding the sale of strong drink in several entire states and in large parts of many other states.

=Tobacco makes the Brain work Slower.=--An examination of the age and habits of hundreds of the students entering a large university in New England showed that those who smoked required more than a year longer than those who did not use tobacco, to learn enough to enter the first classes in this school. Moreover, out of every hundred of those who took the highest rank in their work in the university, ninety-five did not use tobacco. It is likely that tobacco makes the mind work slower by preventing the full amount of blood from going to the brain. It does this by making the blood vessels smaller.

So far as known tobacco has but little effect upon the brains of older persons.

Superintendent Ogg of Indiana reports that the occasional users of cigarettes are a year, and the regular users two years, behind those who do not smoke. The conduct and honesty of the smokers were also found to be lower than among those who did not smoke.

=Opium, Morphine, and Cocaine.=--All of these harmful drugs are widely used in our country. They act on the brain in a strange way. All of them deaden pain. When a person first begins their use, only a small amount is required to produce the effect wanted on the body. Later the doses must be increased. After a few months' use the person becomes a slave to the habit of using them, and he cannot stop their use without the help of a doctor. It is therefore dangerous to use these drugs at any time.

Powders used for colds in the nose, also paregoric and laudanum, contain these harmful drugs.

=Pain Killers and Soothing Sirups.=--All pain killers contain opium or morphine or other harmful drugs. They are therefore dangerous to use. Pain is useful in telling us that some organ is out of order and needs care. Killing the pain does not help the sick organ, and it may let the organ get so sick as to cause death.

One use of the nerves is to tell us when any part of the body is hurt or sick. Pain is nature's warning, and to numb the nerves which tell us about it is as foolish as to kill a person because he brings us bad news. No medicine should ever be given children to make them sleep or stop their crying except by the advice of the physician.

=Powders and Pills.=--If you get sick, do not try to cure yourself with pills or powders bought at the store. Some of these medicines contain poisons which hurt the heart or other organs. A number of persons have been killed by taking such medicines. When you are sick, go to a good doctor who understands how the organs should work, and he will find which one is out of order and tell you exactly what medicine you need and what to eat in order to get well quickly.

=Tea and Coffee.=--These drinks usually wake up the brain and make it work better for a time. If too much of them is used, they may excite the brain in such a way as to make persons nervous. If taken for supper, they may prevent sleep. Children should not use either tea or coffee. Tea sometimes disturbs digestion, and coffee may injure both the stomach and the heart.

PRACTICAL QUESTIONS

1. What is a narcotic?

2. Name some narcotics.

3. What is a stimulant?

4. Name some stimulants.

5. How long before alcohol taken reaches the brain?

6. What effect does strong drink have on the brain?

7. Does alcohol help us think better?

8. What facts show that alcohol sends men to prison?

9. What shows that alcohol makes the mind sick?

10. Why is it dangerous for the young to take strong drink?

11. What shows that tobacco makes the brain work slower?

12. Why should you not use opium or morphine?

13. What do pain killers contain?

CHAPTER XXII

THE SENSES, OR DOORS OF KNOWLEDGE

=The Organs of Sense.=--In order that our body may keep out of the way of other persons and find food and drink and do its work, the brain must have some way of receiving news about what is near us, how it looks, and of what it is made. Special organs for receiving knowledge of people and things about us are scattered over the surface of the body. They are called sense organs. The chief ones are the two eyes, the two ears, the nose, and many organs of taste in the mouth, and the thousands of tiny organs of feeling in the skin.

=The Eye.=--The eye consists of a globe called the eyeball and parts which move this and protect it from injury. Each eyeball is attached at its back part to the large nerve of sight (Fig. 90). This carries messages to the brain, telling it what the eye sees.

The eyeball is held in a socket in the front of the skull. A layer of fat lines the socket and keeps the eye from being injured by jars. The eyebrows at the lower edge of the forehead prevent the sweat from running into the eyeball.

[Illustration: FIG. 90.--Side of the face cut away to show the eyeball in its socket. n is the nerve of sight; the other letters show the muscles which move the eyeball.]

The eyelids can close over the front of the eyeball to shut out dirt or anything else likely to hurt it. The lids have learned to do their work so well that we do not need to think to close them when anything flies toward the eye, for they are shut before we can think.

A salty fluid called tears flows from the tear gland at the upper and outer side of the eyeball. The tears keep the front of the eyeball clean.

=Parts of the Eyeball.=--The outside of the eyeball is a tough white coat except in front, where it is as clear as glass. Within the outer coat is a very thin black lining to keep the light from scattering. In front the lining is not against the outer coat, but hangs loose and has in it a round hole called the pupil to let the light pass through. The part around the hole is the iris. It may be blue, black, or brown, and can squeeze up so as to make the pupil very small when the light is strong.

The end of the nerve of sight forms a tender pink covering over most of the inner surface of the eyeball. The cavity within the eyeball is filled with three clear substances. The lens, shaped like a flat door knob, is fixed just behind the pupil. In front of the lens is a watery fluid and behind it is a clear jellylike mass. The use of the lens and also the other substances is to bend the rays of light together so that they will meet at one place.

=How the Eyeball is Moved.=--Six muscles fixed to the bones of the socket holding the eye have their other ends fastened to the tough coat of the eyeball. One muscle turns the ball upward, another turns it downward, one turns it inward and another turns it outward. If an inner or an outer muscle is too strong, a person may have cross eyes.

=Keeping the Eye Strong.=--Nearly all young children have perfect eyes. After a year or two in school the eyes of some children become weak. Many children get weak eyes after they are ten or twelve years old. This is because they have not taken care of the eyes.

The eyes are often hurt by reading a book with fine print, reading in a dim light, or by leaning over the book so that the eyes look downward instead of straight forward. As the eyes are very weak after measles and most other diseases, they should not be used much until a week or more after recovery.

In reading the book should be held a little over a foot in front of the chest and you should sit nearly straight and let the light fall on the page from one side. Never read while lying down because it strains the eyes. Stop reading as soon as the eyes smart.

=Helping the Eyes to See.=--Very few old people can see to read without the help of glasses, because the lens of the eye hardens in old age. To see things near by, the shape of the lens must be changed. In some children, the shape of the eyes has become so changed by straining them to read fine print or see things in a dim light that the eyes hurt after being used for any kind of work, and the head may often ache and make the whole body feel bad. Such eyes need help. You should have them examined by an eye doctor who can fit you with glasses which will help you see clearly without headache.

=Keeping the Eyes Well.=--Bits of dirt often get beneath the eyelids and cause much pain. By taking hold of the eyelashes the lid may be pulled out from the eye and any dirt removed with the corner of a clean handkerchief passed gently along the lid.

The eyes sometimes become sore because they are rubbed with soiled fingers on which are germs. These germs get inside the lids and grow, and in this way poison the eyes. Unless care is used sore eyes are likely to spread from one child to another in the school. The sick child rubs its eyes and then handles a book or pencil on which the germs are smeared by the fingers which touched the eyes. The next child picks up the same book later, gets the germs on the fingers, and then rubs the eyes. For this reason you should never rub the eyes. If you have sore eyes, be careful that no one else catches the sickness from you.

=The Ear.=--The ear is made of three parts called the outer ear, the middle ear or eardrum, and the inner ear. The outer ear is made of a plate of skin and gristle and a slightly bent tube about one inch long. At the inner end of this tube is a thin membrane or drumhead. Beyond the drumhead is the cavity of the middle ear about as large as a pea. A chain of three tiny bones stretches from the outer drumhead across this cavity to a tiny inner drumhead. Beyond the inner drumhead is the inner ear.

The middle ear is kept full of air by means of a tube leading from it to the throat. A cold or other sickness may cause this tube to fill up and make you deaf. The inner ear consists of a sac and four bent tubes filled with a watery fluid. They are also surrounded by watery fluid contained in channels in a bone of the skull. The end of the nerve of hearing is on one of the tubes.

=How we Hear.=--Throwing a stone in the water makes waves which move farther and farther outward. In the same way a noise causes waves in the air. These waves pass into the ear tube, strike the outer drumhead, and make it move. This moves the chain of bones in the middle ear so that they cause motion in the inner drumhead. This in moving back and forth makes waves in the fluid of the inner ear which strike on the ends of the nerve of hearing and cause messages to be carried to the brain.

=Care of the Ears.=--The ears should not be struck or pulled, as the eardrum is easily broken. Do not put pencils, pins, or anything else in your ears. Wax naturally forms in the ear tube to keep out bugs and flies. The outer part of the tube may be kept clean by wiping it with a moist cloth over the little finger. If you often have earache or a running ear, you should have it examined by a physician. Neglecting a sick ear may cause deafness.

Some persons are deaf in one ear and do not know it. Test each ear by covering the other one with a heavy cloth and note how far off you can hear the ticks of a watch.

=The Nose.=--The nose has a skin-like lining, but it is always kept moist by little glands which give out a watery fluid. The endings of the nerve of smell are in the lining in the upper part of the nose. Two nerves lead from the nose to the brain.

When we catch cold, much blood rushes to the lining of the nose and it becomes swollen. It then gives out a thick white mucus. This covers the nerve endings, so that we cannot smell.

Smell is of great use in telling us whether our food is good, by helping us to enjoy food with a pleasant odor, and by warning us against bad air.

=The Sense of Taste.=--The nerves by which we taste end in the soft covering of the tongue and some other parts of the mouth. A food cannot be tasted while it is dry. For this reason much slippery fluid flows into the mouth from glands under the ears and tongue. This fluid, called saliva, softens the solid food when it is well chewed, so we can taste it.

=The Senses of the Skin.=--There are endings of nerves in the skin all over the body. They are of three or four different kinds. Some of them tell us about heat, others tell us about cold. Some tell us about the shape, the smoothness, or hardness of objects, while others tell us when the skin gets hurt.

Most of the nerve endings are in the deeper part of the skin, so that they are covered by the epidermis and cannot be hurt by the rough things handled.

=Alcohol and the Senses.=--The senses are but little affected by a small amount of alcoholic drink. The sense of taste, after being accustomed to the sharpness of strong drink, may be less easily pleased with the taste of common food and drink.

The use of large amounts of alcohol blunts all the senses. In a drunken man the senses of the skin are so numbed that he does not know when anything touches him, and he may be badly burned before he feels the pain.

Heavy drinking makes the hearing less keen, enlarges the blood vessels of the eyes, and makes them appear red and bloodshot.

=Tobacco and the Senses.=--The use of tobacco does not injure the senses of the skin and usually has no effect on hearing. Both chewing and smoking, if much practiced, make the sense of taste less delicate, so that one cannot enjoy his food to the fullest extent.

Much smoking of tobacco may hurt the nerve of sight and in a few cases it has made men blind. Many boys have weakened their eyes by the use of cigarettes.

PRACTICAL QUESTIONS

1. Name the chief sense organs.

2. Of what use are the eyelids and tears?

3. Name four parts of the eyeball.

4. What is the iris?

5. Of what use is the lens?

6. What moves the eyeball?

7. When do children get weak eyes?

8. How are the eyes often hurt?

9. How may poor eyes be helped?

10. What makes the eyes sore?

11. How do germs get into the eyes?

12. Name the three parts of the ear.

13. What does the inner ear contain?

14. What may result from neglecting a sick ear?

15. Of what use is smell?

16. Why should food be well chewed?

17. In what part of the skin are most of the nerve endings?

18. What effect does tobacco have on the sense of taste?

CHAPTER XXIII

KEEPING AWAY SICKNESS

=Too Much Sickness.=--Many diseases are caused by our own carelessness and our bad habits of living. We have about one doctor for every one hundred families. There are enough people sick every day to make a city as large as New York or to equal the number of people living in the thirteen states of Idaho, Nevada, Wyoming, Arizona, New Mexico, Utah, Delaware, Montana, Vermont, New Hampshire, North Dakota and South Dakota, and Oklahoma.

A careful study of disease and its cause shows that at least one half of all the sickness in our land can be avoided by right living.

=The Cause of Sickness.=--Some people are so foolish as to make themselves sick. They weaken the body by using much beer or wine, by breathing bad air, by lack of exercise, or by fast eating. When the body becomes weak, it is likely to get sick at any time.

It is not always our own fault when we are sick. It may be caused by the carelessness of others who have let germs escape from their bodies so that they are able to reach us. One half of the sickness in our land is catching sickness. That is, it is sickness which passes from one person to another and is caused by tiny germs or microbes. A catching sickness is called a contagious disease. Some of the common catching diseases are sore throat, colds, diphtheria, pneumonia, typhoid fever, measles, grippe, and whooping cough.

=How we get a Catching Sickness.=--We get a catching sickness by taking into our bodies the germs from some other person. The germs of the sick do not pass off in the breath, but in the spit or anything else which comes from their bodies. This is why the spit and all slops from the sick room should be burned, buried, or destroyed in some way.

[Illustration: FIG. 94.--How the germs of disease start on their mission of death. This sewer carries slops from the houses of the sick and well and empties into a stream used below for drinking water.]

We should think it very wicked if a showman should turn his lions and tigers loose in a crowd of women and children. Somebody would surely be killed and others hurt. It is just as wrong to turn loose the germs of the sick by throwing the spit and the slops where they will get into a stream or where the flies may find them and by soiling their feet leave death in their trail wherever they crawl.

=How the Germs of Sickness catch Us.=--The germs of sickness have no feet to walk and no wings to fly, yet they easily travel from the sick to the well. They are not killed by being frozen, or drowned by floating in water, or destroyed by drying. For this reason they can travel with the ice, water, milk, and dust.

In Buffalo, New York, fifty-seven children caught the scarlet fever in one week by using milk cared for by a boy who was getting well from the scarlet fever.

The germs of sickness are so small that a million can hang to the hands or clothing and not be seen. For this reason they are often left clinging to the fingers, desks, books, and pencils, and travel in large numbers on the feet of flies. The surest way the germs have of getting from one person to another is by the common drinking cup.

[Illustration: FIG. 95.--Photograph of clear beef broth jelly in which a fly walked five minutes scattering germs. Two days later each germ brushed off the fly's feet grew into a city of germs appearing as a white spot.]

=The Common Drinking Cup is an Exchange Station for Germs.=--The most careful examinations have shown that there are thousands of children as well as grown persons who have very light attacks of scarlet fever, tuberculosis, or other diseases and go to school or about their work scattering the germs of sickness in their spit. A child seldom drinks from a cup without leaving on it thousands of germs. Some of these may be germs which will cause sickness. On one drinking cup used in a school, the germs were found to be as thick as the leaves on a maple tree in June.

In an Ohio school one warm day, a boy with beginning measles drank from the cup which was afterward used on the same day by the teacher and all the other pupils. In less than two weeks every pupil and the teacher were suffering from measles. Put nothing into your mouth which has been in another's mouth.

=The Golden Rule.=--If you have a catching sickness, such as measles, chicken pox, or whooping cough, stay away from others. Since the germs of some diseases, like scarlet fever and diphtheria, remain in the spit sometimes several months after you feel well, don't scatter your spit. Hold a handkerchief before your face when you sneeze or cough. Wash your hands before handling food.

=Some Animals carry Sickness.=--Mosquitoes carry malaria and yellow fever and some other diseases. Flies carry typhoid fever, grippe, diphtheria, and tuberculosis. Bedbugs and fleas carry the plague and leprosy. Rats carry the plague. Cats sometimes carry diphtheria. Many cows have tuberculosis and the germs of this disease are then sometimes found in their milk. Some children have caught tuberculosis from drinking such milk.

=Keeping away Smallpox.=--Smallpox was once the most terrible of all diseases. It is so catching that two or three were often sick with it at one time in the same family. Sometimes nearly one half the people of a whole town would have the disease in one year. Over a hundred years ago nearly every grown up person had little pits scattered over his face as a result of having had smallpox.

You can always keep away smallpox by being vaccinated. The doctor can vaccinate you by putting on the freshly scraped skin of your arm some weak smallpox germs from a clean healthy calf which has been vaccinated. Your arm will in a few days get sore and you will not feel well for about one week, but you will be made safe from smallpox for several years.

Fifty nurses were vaccinated in Philadelphia and cared for many sick with the smallpox, staying with them day after day, but not one of the nurses took the disease. Every one should be vaccinated when a year old and again at the age of ten or twelve years.

=Colds.=--Some colds are catching, but we generally take cold because we have weak bodies or have been careless. If you want to be free from colds, remember these six rules:--

Don't sit still in wet clothes or with wet feet.

Don't sit in a cold draft or in a cold room.

Don't sit on the damp ground or on the ice when you are resting from skating.

Don't cool off quickly after exercising.

Sleep in a room with the windows wide open.

Take a cold bath every morning and draw fresh air to the bottom of the lungs many times every day.

=Tuberculosis or Consumption.=--This disease is so common and deadly that twenty persons die from it in our country every hour. It is caused by tiny germs (Fig. 63) which lodge in the lungs, glands, bones, or other parts of the body, where they give off poison and hurt the tissues. We take these germs into the body with dust or food, and also by putting to the lips a drinking cup or other things used by a consumptive. Generally the germs will not grow in a strong body, even when they have lodged there.

=Preventing Consumption.=--Living in poorly lighted houses without much fresh air, working in dusty rooms, using much strong drink and tobacco, eating poor food, losing sleep, neglecting a cough, and taking little or no outdoor exercise weaken the body so that the consumption germs can grow in it. Deep breathing, sitting and walking erect, living in rooms with sunshine, sleeping with the windows open eight or nine hours every night, and eating good food will prevent one from taking consumption and will often cure the disease. Persons with this sickness give out the germs in their spit, which should be caught in a cup and burned.

=The Hookworm Disease.=--This is a sickness affecting thousands of persons in the South. It is caused by tiny worms half as large as a pin hanging fast to the lining of the bowels. The worm is sometimes called the lazy germ because it destroys the red blood cells and makes the body feel weak and lazy. Children with these worms grow slowly, have a dry skin, and a swollen abdomen with a tender spot below the stomach.

The disease is easily cured by a physician, but it is better to prevent it by killing the germs in the waste from the bowels. For directions, address the Department of Health at the capital of your state. If the germs reach the ground they crawl around and may get into the well, and enter the body again with the drinking water. Generally, however, the worms enter through the skin of those going barefooted, and are carried by the blood to the lungs. From here they go up the windpipe to the throat, and then down the gullet to the bowels. It is their entrance through the skin that causes ground itch or dew itch. Wearing shoes will help prevent the disease.

=A Strong Body Wins.=--Nobody wants to be weak and sickly. Most all of us could keep well if we would try in the right way to keep the body strong.

To keep the body in health it must have plenty of sleep, enough good food well chewed, plenty of clean water, exercise every day, and an abundance of fresh air. The body is the temple of the soul. Don't hurt it with bad habits.

PRACTICAL QUESTIONS

1. How many people are sick to-day in our country?

2. How can much sickness be avoided?

3. What causes sickness?

4. What is a contagious disease?

5. Name some contagious diseases.

6. How do we get a catching sickness?

7. Why should we be careful with the slops from the sick room?

8. Tell how children in Buffalo caught scarlet fever.

9. What is the danger in using a cup from which others have drunk?

10. How can you prevent others from getting your sickness?

11. Name some animals which carry sickness.

12. How can we keep away smallpox?

13. Give six rules to keep away colds.

14. How may the body be kept strong?

CHAPTER XXIV

HELPING BEFORE THE DOCTOR COMES

=The Need of Quick Help.=--In many places in the country, or when out camping, it is impossible to get a doctor in less than two or three hours. Unless some one at hand can give aid before the doctor comes, much suffering and even death may result when a simple accident occurs. For this reason every one should know how to help in case of such accidents as burns, bleeding, choking, and sunstroke.

=Clothing on Fire.=--Children should never play about an open fire. A single spark lighting on a cotton dress may cause it to burst into a blaze so that within a few minutes the child is enveloped in flames.

The quickest way to put out such a fire is to wrap the child in a blanket, a piece of carpet, a coat, or any part of your clothing quickly removed. If nothing is at hand to wrap the sufferer in, roll him over and over in the dirt or weeds until the flames are smothered. When your clothing is on fire, you must not run, because this fans the fire and makes it burn.

=Burns and Scalds.=--If there is clothing on the part burned, it should be taken off slowly so as not to tear the skin. If the clothing sticks, soak it in oil a few minutes until it gets loose. Cover the burned part as quickly as possible with vaseline or a clean cloth soaked in a quart of boiled water containing a cup of washing soda. Let nothing dirty touch the burned surface and keep it well wrapped.

=Bleeding.=--A person can lose a quart of blood without danger of death and may live after more than two quarts have been lost, but it is wise to try to stop any flow of blood as quickly as possible. Tying a clean cloth folded several times over the cut will in most cases stop the flow. This will help a clot to form and will also close the ends of the cut vessels if the bandage is twisted tight with a stick.

If the cut is on a limb and the blood comes out in spurts, a bandage tied about the limb between the cut and the body may be twisted tight with a stick so as to press upon the artery and close it. A piece of wood or folded cloth placed over the artery under the bandage before it is tightened is helpful.

=Nosebleed.=--Some persons are troubled frequently with bleeding from the nose. The least knock may cause it to bleed for more than an hour. It may generally be stopped without sending for a doctor.

Sit up straight to keep the blood out of the head and press the middle part of the nose firmly between the fingers. Apply a cold wet cloth or a lump of ice wrapped in a cloth to the back of the neck. Put a bag of pounded ice on the root of the nose. If it does not stop in a half hour, wet a soft rag or a piece of cotton with cold tea or alum water and put it gently into the bleeding nostril so as to entirely close it. Do not blow the nose for several hours after the bleeding has stopped as this may start it again.

=Fainting.=---Fainting may be caused by bad air, an overheated room, by fear, or by some other excitement. A fainting person falls down and appears to be asleep. The lips are pale and there may be cold sweat on the forehead. There is too little blood in the brain, and the heart is weak.

A fainting person should be laid flat on the floor or on a couch, and all doors and windows opened wide. Loosen all tight clothing and apply to the forehead a cloth wet with cold water. A faint usually lasts only a few minutes.

=Sunstroke.=---A person with sunstroke becomes giddy, sick at the stomach, and weak. He then gets drowsy and may seem as if asleep, but he cannot be aroused. The skin is hot and dry instead of being cold and pale, as in fainting. The doctor should be sent for at once.

The first aid for sunstroke is to put the patient in a cool cellar or an icehouse, raise the head, and wet the head, neck, and back of the chest with cold water. As soon as he wakens put him in a cool room.

=Frostbite.=---When out in very cold weather, the end of the nose, the tips of the ears, and the toes and fingers are sometimes frozen. If a person comes into a warm room, these frozen parts will give much pain. The parts should be rubbed with snow or ice water until a tingling sensation is felt.

=Breaks in the Skin.=---A small cut or tear in the skin may become very sore and cause much trouble if not cared for so as to keep the germs out. If there is dirt in the wound, as when made with a rusty nail or by the bite of a dog, it should be squeezed and washed with boiled water to make it perfectly clean. It may then be bound up in a clean cloth. A little turpentine poured on the wound will help kill the germs which may make it sore. If the dog is thought to be mad or the wound is too deep to be easily washed out to the bottom, a doctor should be called.

=Snakebite.=---The scratches made by the little teeth of most snakes, such as the milk snake, garter snake, and black snake, do no more harm than the scratch of a pin. The copperhead, the southern moccasin, and the rattlesnake have a pair of long teeth called fangs in the upper jaw. These teeth have little canals in them through which the snake presses poison into the bite.

If a person is bitten by one of these snakes, the doctor must be sent for and help given at once. Put a bandage above the bite and twist it tight with a stick. Make two or three deep cuts into the bitten place to let out the poisoned blood. Suck the wound to draw out the poison and apply ammonia.

=Choking.=--A hard piece of meat, a bone, or a peach seed may slip back into the throat and press so hard on the windpipe as to cut off the air from the lungs. If the object is not far back in the throat, it may be seized with the first finger. A few smart slaps on the upper part of the back while the body is bent forward may drive enough air out of the lungs to push the object outward.

=Drowning.=--Every one should learn to swim while young, but no one should venture in deep water. Stiffening of the muscles called cramps often causes the best swimmer to drown.

After a person has been under the water two or three minutes he appears lifeless. He may, however, be brought to life if laid face downward, his clothes loosened, and the lungs made to breathe. A heavy folded coat, a piece of sod, or a bunch of weeds should be put under the chest. Then standing astride of him place the hands on the lower ribs and bend forward gradually so as to press on the ribs and push the air out of the lungs. Then straighten your body and slowly lessen pressure on the patient's ribs so that the air will run into the lungs. In this way make the air go in and out of the lungs about fifteen times each minute.

=Poisoning.=--Whenever a person has taken poison, a physician should be sent for at once. In most cases an effort should be made to get the poison out of the stomach by causing vomiting. A glass or two of weak, warm soapsuds, a pint of water with a tablespoonful of mustard, or a glass of water with two tablespoonfuls of salt may be taken to make the stomach throw out the poison. Tickling the throat back of the tongue will help cause vomiting.

If a strong acid such as carbolic acid or a strong alkali such as ammonia has been taken, do not cause vomiting. For acids give chalk in warm water and a pint of milk. For an alkali give vinegar in water.

###